Eyesight

Strengthen Your Vision the Natural Way

(How to Strengthen Your Eye Muscles and to Improve Your Vision)

Matthew Peraza

Published By **Kate Sanders**

Matthew Peraza

Eyesight: Strengthen Your Vision the Natural Way (How to Strengthen Your Eye Muscles and to Improve Your Vision)

ISBN   978-1-7780063-7-1

No part of this guidebook shall be reproduced in any form without permission in writing from the publisher except in the case of brief quotations embodied in critical articles or reviews.

Legal & Disclaimer

The information contained in this book is not designed to replace or take the place of any form of medicine or professional medical advice. The information in this book has been provided for educational & entertainment purposes only.

The information contained in this book has been compiled from sources deemed reliable, and it is accurate to the best of the Author's knowledge; however, the Author cannot guarantee its accuracy and validity and cannot be held liable for any errors or omissions. Changes are periodically made to this book. You must consult your doctor or get professional medical advice before using any of the suggested remedies, techniques, or information in this book.

Table Of Contents

Chapter 1: You Will Require Glasses 1

Chapter 2: I'm A Myope 7

Chapter 3: Common Treatment 23

Chapter 4: Do You Really Require Glasses?
.... 33

Chapter 5: Finding The Solution 47

Chapter 6: A Dramatic Improvements.... 57

Chapter 7: Manage Your Expectations ... 74

Chapter 8: There Are No Tools That You
Require Are The Tools You 81

Chapter 9: What Can You Do To Increase
Your Distance Vision 97

Chapter 10: Good Habits For Vision 116

Chapter 11: Prevention 122

Chapter 12: A The Nearsighted Crisis ... 133

Chapter 13: The Nearsighted Eye Doctor
.... 145

Chapter 14: The Essential Habits For Optimal Eye Health 153

Chapter 15: The Critical Eye Companions 164

Chapter 16: Work With You're Vision Therapy Coach Along With You............ 175

Chapter 1: You Will Require Glasses

At some point between 11 and 12, I was required to purchase glasses. I was adamant about wearing glasses. they were too stupid They didn't look good on my face and got filthy too easily and also hindered my ability to participate in the activities I had always wanted to do outdoors such as playing soccer and skateboarding.

It was impossible to wake up and do what I wanted because the first thing I saw every morning was a blurry, but recognizable picture from my room. The glasses proved to be a major issue for me, and I was dissatisfied that I had change my routine in order to make room for glasses. I didn't realize in such a short time that I'd need to keep wearing the glasses.

How do I obtain glasses?

I remember vividly the tests for hearing and vision which are administered to children in the middle of elementary school. These tests are vital for determining if there are any difficulties as children get older and develop, the examination for vision will often be an obvious sign that a child is likely to struggle to read the whiteboard. As with many kids my age, I was unable to be doing very well in the test of vision.

When I was told of my poor vision My parents took me to an optometrist who recommended an amount of correction to aid me in seeing better when I was in the classroom. It's not clear if I should be congratulating myself. were appropriate, but it appears I'm now successfully treated!

When I was a child I would spend all in the outdoors. I did everything outdoors. I was not really wanting to go inside since, truthfully, there wasn't many things to do other than watching TV.

If we look back, watching television likely not be the ideal choice for development. Do you remember the times that your parents told that you shouldn't sit near to the TV to ensure that you didn't damage your eyesight? It could have had some truth in the advice.

There I was. A child who spends so much time outdoors and was suddenly unexpectedly required to wear glasses in order so that he could see and read better in class. If you're familiar with this and it's not a surprise as it was the reason we all started to wear glasses.

This isn't really remarkable, especially given that it is during this time that the majority of kids are locked in their rooms for long periods of time in dark classrooms. They are battling to draw small letters on whiteboards.

I don't recall the bright fluorescent lamps in the classrooms as being especially brilliant. In comparison to sunlight in the natural environment this is like living in a dark space. They are one of the most unsuitable types to be used everywhere. They emit a sour hue of light that just create a situation that is hard to comprehend. Was it truly my fault that I was unable to read well enough?

Glasses were not a good idea for me or any other kid who was active and enjoyed spending time outside. I was so disappointed that I was unable to be able to see clearly enough in school Maybe I should have stayed clear of glasses all together.

Most people wearing contacts or glasses had the same experiences that I had. It is possible that there are some that started wearing glasses following becoming adults. I would guess they required them following having started working at a cubicle farm, or an indoor work space with a similar lack of lighting.

It is then that everyone gets comfortable wearing the glasses and then being dependent on glasses. What's the very initial thing that you'll do after you wake up? It's putting on your glasses so you're able to clearly see before you begin your day. Each day.

I sure did. So did millions of people. The glasses were provided to us and did not receive any instructions on how to use them properly.

In some way I was under the belief that I needed to wear glasses every day. I didn't remember receiving any particular advice from an optometrist about exactly how and when to wear glasses. Was I aware that I shouldn't utilize these devices when I was reading from a distance? There was no instructions on the proper usage of these dangerous devices.

Following the first prescribed, that ranged between -2.0 to -3.0 diopters, I began wearing them throughout the course throughout the day. In coincidentally, I began experiencing severe headaches. The first couple of weeks were terrible. The headaches would come and go until my eyes quit from fighting. The doctor told me it was normal. Looking back, it appears as if my body was telling me something was not right.

For me, it was a bad experience because I was required to wear glasses. It all started with the time I was required to wear glasses to school.

Chapter 2: I'm A Myope

The reality is that if you're unable to clearly see in the distance, you might are suffering from a condition known as myopia.

What exactly is myopia?

Before the topic, let's examine various parts that make up the eye, and their functions:

Cornea - the front of the eye which reflects light. It can be capable of absorbing up to two thirds of refractive powers of the eye.

Lens is a transparent device which alters its length in order so that it can focus images on the retina. Lenses can be capable of sustaining up to one third the power of an eye

Ciliary body controls the form of the lens in order to be focused on close or distant things

Retina is a light-sensitive cell within the eye that converts the visible world into an image for the brain.

Pupil is the opening of the eye which allows certain amounts of light to reflect off the rear of the retina.

Each of these elements work in order to focus the eye on a variety of objects of different distances. They cooperate so that the eye can rapidly focus on anything that is just one foot away to more than 100 feet.

First, let's look at the normal eye and see how light is received and viewed. The normal eye is where light passes through the cornea. It then travels through the lens. The lens is controlled by the body of the ciliary. It brings the image to focus, which is reflected on the retina.

In this image, we can clearly see that light is passing through the lens and cornea. Since the image is reflected to the rear of the retina, and it is focused, the size as well as the shape of the eyeball is normal. Eyes with this shape are likely to be able to be able to see clearly even at long distances. The image will never be blurred.

What happens when identical images at the same distance is projected by an eyeball that is physically extended?

The image reflects onto the retina because of the lengthening of our eyes. The result is blurred images. All objectives that are viewed over the specified distance will be blurred. For this reason it is necessary to use a corrective lens. like eyeglasses or contact lenses should be placed directly in front of the cornea in order to be capable of seeing clearly.

If you've used an camera that has manually adjusted focus, then you can imagine that you shift the lens. The lens' components are moved closer or farther away, bringing the image to the focus.

The various components of the eye function similarly. The lens, ciliary organ as well as the cornea carry out majority of the heavy lifting so that you can concentrate on distant and close things. They also have inherent boundaries. In cases where the whole length the eyes has changed through time, the various parts of the eyes struggle to create a clear picture.

We get close to the definition

Nearsightedness, also known as myopia, is a condition that occurs when it is possible to see objects near quite clearly. However, distant objects seem blurred.

The shape of the eyes causes the rays of light to bend towards the retina rather than directly to the retina. This results in a blurred image in the event of viewing something from the distance. In order to correct this issue it is necessary to reduce the length of your eye must be shortened to a level in which the image concentrates to the retina rather than directly in front.

We now know the causes of myopia It is important to know what is the cause of it.

How did you develop myopia?

Did you ever remember being a child and you sat for all day in the classroom? You read a variety of textbooks as well as doing lots of work in your workstation. A majority of these tasks were performed at close ranges that were less than an arm's distance. Reading in close proximity over the course of several years in a row, you did irreparable damage to your vision distance. It led to the need for correction lenses as a child. age.

To understand the relationship to better understand this connection, researchers from the Sydney Myopia Study collected data between 2004 and the year 2005 for an over-2,000 Australian students between 12 and 13 years old. This study looked into the amount of time spending outdoors as well as indoors every day. They also measured the amount of time read.

The research found that there's the direct connection between being able to read up close (defined to be within 30cm which is about 12 inches) over a long period of duration (over 30 mins) as well as the higher risk of developing myopia among youngsters. [1]

In simple terms, it is the case if you read in close proximity for long periods of time and your vision for distance is likely to diminish. Any similar activity that is close to you can cause the same effect as well as lead to myopia. We can also refer to this kind of reading close work.

When I picture the classroom, and I imagine kids at their desks, I notice that the books placed on the desks don't sit closer than the distance of 30 centimeters from their pupils. This probably isn't a thought to the majority of individuals that there's something that is wrong.

It is a fact that children across the globe spend a large majority of their time reading in the indoors. Classrooms are a great space that gives children an opportunity to think, learn and discover. However. It is now evident that there's a danger for eyesight damage if this kind of work in close proximity is carried out for a prolonged period. However, I've not received any warnings concerning this kind of practice at the schools, at universities or even from teachers and parents.

What are other causes of myopia?

If children are beginning to develop poor habits like working in the vicinity of work for long hours each day, their eyesight deteriorates rapidly, and suddenly they're required to have vision correction. Since they've been experiencing problems reading whiteboards and composing their thoughts, they now have prescription corrective or minus, lenses. These come with a power rating that is stated as a negative diopter like -1.0 or -2.75 or any other value that is negative. The students must use these lenses on a regular basis for the duration of their time in the classroom.

If you're not aware of the concept diopter, it's a measurement unit for the lens's optical performance. A 4 diopter lens will bring rays light into focus at the equivalent of 1/4 of an inch. In the same way, a two diopter lens can do exactly the same thing at 1/2 of an inch.

Sadly, when many people wear lenses that are corrective and use lenses for work in close proximity the eyesight is beginning to become worse. The reason for this is that they were originally designed to permit the wearer to look at faraway objects. There is not a reason why they should be used in situations where something can be observed clearly from a distance, and without correction.

However, what are the most common things people do? If they have to wear contact lenses or glasses, they'll probably wear them throughout the throughout the day. It's difficult to get them removed for working, specifically when wearing contact lenses.

So, the gradual and evident decline in distance vision happens over the course of time. The eyeball grows physically in size and length while it attempts to adjust to seeing the world without lenses. Vision that is already weak needs stronger and stronger prescription lenses as time passes. The result is an ongoing loop, which can cause eyesight to become worse as time passes. Some people can continue for a long time, while for other people, it'll stop in a particular level.

Myopia is a term that can be summarized as progressing with time and in these circumstances.

Excessive reading of the books or screens including tablets and computers when at a close distance or in dim lighting

Extensive periods of near working cause the eyes to grow longer, and they now require corrective glasses to read at the same distance.

Work continues near to home following the use of corrective lenses. closer distances, which makes the eye grow larger.

A further decline in vision will require stronger and more lens and this process is repeated.

What did my optometrist not tell me about my alternatives?

Optometrists' main function is to give you the most effective treatment for the current issue with your vision. It is their goal to provide patients with treatment but it is not always a means of treatment.

One of the most efficient ways to achieve it is to supply the corrective lenses you need to let you see clearly in the distance. Most customers prefer a speedy option, not a solution that involves a substantial amount of time and dedication.

I'm not certain if optometrists even want to advocate alternative solutions even if they knew of these. Do they really have a business case for them to suggest against contacts or glasses?

The purpose of this book is not to explore the reason what causes prevention strategies don't seem to be being used more often. The reason it's not considered widely known could stem from human nature. Humans tend to be lazy and possess the tendency to want immediate satisfaction. If someone has poor distance vision, the fastest and most effective method to address their issues is to purchase glasses that let them be able to see clearly and immediately. To accomplish this, an optometrist can be a useful resource.

There's a lot of money available for purchasing eyeglasses as well as to cover vision tests. There's an entire field that is dedicated to a clear vision I'll blame it on those who are unaware that other solutions are available.

Is it possible to reverse myopia?

Reversing the myopia-related process isn't easy. There are numerous unsuccessful and unstudied strategies that I've come across during my studies. I've come across "eye exercises" that instruct the user to gaze across the sides or upwards and downwards in order to strengthen muscles in the eye that move. There are no research that supports the claimed positive effects of these exercises.

I've not come across any sort of official or government-backed information on the treatment of myopia. The science-based resources can be difficult to discern whether there's a cure for myopia.

If you go online to find the definition of and treatments for myopia, a lot of medical websites will only tell you what treatment options are available. This treatment includes glasses that correct the vision or undergo laser surgery. Although surgery is generally considered risk-free, it's an operation that is still risky and comes with risks.

There are very limited resources on reverse the damage caused by this process to your eyesight. How come it is so difficult to discover? The reason is that the procedure to reverse myopia understood more widely when we understand the root causes?

The most straightforward way to reverse myopia is to not wear prescription lenses in circumstances where they're not required. Do you really have to use corrective lenses for scrolling your phone in a close proximity? No, definitely not.

Minus lenses are intended to let you see distant objects or texts and are best used in the circumstances. Do you think that you would use the binoculars you have to view the television?

The majority of people wear them without even a second thought in all routine actions. In fact, it is the continual wearing of these lenses close work which causes the progression of myopia.

In the course of years of continual utilization of corrective lenses in any work that is both close and far The ciliary muscle that is responsible for focusing the lens gets stretched to the limits of its ability. Though more research must be carried out in this area this could lead to the reason why the prescription prescribed for most adults seems to be stable within a certain diopter.

This is referred to as a spasm or accommodation or an subciliary spasm. The muscle stays constantly in contraction, and it is no longer functioning in the way it was intended to. When you've suffered so much injury and strain, it is extremely difficult to get rid of corrective lenses as you've developed a dependence on these lenses. If you do not wear the lenses, everything becomes an illusion.

What could I do to improve my blurred vision?

Once we've got an understanding of the way the eye functions, why the eyes have weakened over the years, and why it is continuing to grow in length We can then look at various common methods of treatment. In a subsequent section, we'll examine certain evidences that help clarify why certain methods in this book effectively prevent and reverse myopia, and enable the ciliary muscles to restore its function.

Chapter 3: Common Treatment

In the course of your life, I'm certain you've been through the bustling center. What's hilarious? It is almost a certain likelihood of finding a retailer with eyeglasses and shades from wall-to-wall. Additionally, they usually will also provide the services of an optometrist who conducts a vision test prior to drafting you an eyeglass prescription that can be used for traditional glasses as well as contact lenses or both.

Many will even give the prescription lenses you need to be custom-ground within a single hour after the time you visit. You could quickly walk into the store to receive an updated prescription, then order glasses as you stroll around the shopping mall as you wait for your new glasses to arrive and delivered within two hours.

I've used this kind of service and, as I mentioned in the book, these services can be beneficial because they permit people who have poor vision distance to swiftly solve their problem by purchasing a brand new pair of spectacles that allow users to see clearly. It's very easy and cost-effective.

Treatment 1: Eyeglasses

The most popular solution for myopes is simply a pair of spectacles without lenses. They are able to be ordered custom and ground in-store to fit your prescription. Many find it an excellent option.

Benefits:

Easy to use

Very easy to clean

Frame design and color selections

Disadvantages:

High cost, even when you have vision insurance

It is essential to clean the lens regularly to keep smudges and oil and dirt from building up on lenses.

Might not be suitable for physical activities like sports.

The risk of scratching and damage when dropped

Contact lenses are the simplest option of all. They can be used by most with the added feature of not causing irritation in the eye as could be common with contact lenses.

They're also the most cost-effective treatment for myopia. Frames with higher quality can be costly, however they are something that you do not need to purchase regularly.

The ease and accessibility of locations to purchase eyeglasses is an enormous benefit of this treatment. But, what are the disadvantages? Most insurance companies only provide coverage for one frame and lenses per calendar year. Additionally, upgrades to lenses including anti-reflective and anti-scratch coatings aren't always covered within the protection and may add cost.

If you are physically active, glasses may not be the ideal solution. It's not pleasant having a pair frames that bounce around your face while you run, jog or engage in any other activity. Do you expect to sweat? Also, your glasses should be. They are a minor inconvenience that diminishes the advantages from wearing glasses. There is no reason to be surprised that those with these issues tend to prefer contact lenses.

Treatment 2: Contact Lenses

Contact lenses provide more flexibility than spectacles, as they provide an appearance that resembles normal vision but do not have to put on frames.

Benefits:

The appearance of normal vision without frames or any other object blocking the face or field of vision

Available for daily disposable options or in longer-term versions

There's no cleaning required to dispose of the versions.

Allows for vigorous physical exercise

Disadvantages:

More expensive when than traditional glasses

Contacts designed for multiple weeks of use must be cleaned regularly using products that add to the total cost

Can be difficult to wear and might not stay on the correct position throughout the whole day

Could cause significant dry eye, or any other irritated

The primary benefits of wearing contact lenses is that they're similar to having no glasses whatsoever. They are not uncomfortable to wear. lenses if they are applied properly. It is not a frame for example, eyeglasses which offer a clear, sharp view ahead, however a blurred line on the other side of the view. It is not a risk of being covered in sweat, or being scratched or damaged. Most of the time they are held in place effectively.

What are the negatives of contact lenses? One of the main issues is price. It is possible to choose from two weeks, a month, or a daily disposable. They come in a range of styles, brands colours, as well as prices. If you opt for a disposable option, you'll typically pay more. There is the convenience of not needing to clean lenses after each day's usage is a factor. If you choose to utilize an extended period of time or another model of lens, there are additional expenses in cleaning products and the time needed to integrate the lenses to your daily routine.

If you wear cosmetics, like mascara on their eyelids, contact lenses may cause severe irritation. In the process of applying different kinds of cosmetics, you may accidently apply too much to your eyelid, and it comes in contact with the lens and can result in uncomfortable irritation. After that, it is necessary to remove the lens and replace it into.

Although contact lenses are a great option and suitable for active people, there is an alternative solution that is available for a higher expense.

Treatment 3: Laser surgery

Laser eye surgery comes with a range of options, which include the LASIK (laser assisted in-situ Keratomileusis) and PRK (photorefractive Keratectomy) and LASEK (laser epithelial Keratomileusis). Every one of them has distinct advantages and disadvantages, and the best procedure for you will depend on the individual's eye state and their years of age.

Benefits:

Based on the kind of surgery performed, lasers is a simple procedure

Provides a permanent, clear and unobstructed view (unless you require touch ups)

Allows you to returning to normal activities with no any significant time to recover

Disadvantages:

Not every person is the perfect candidate for surgery.

May require a lengthy period of recovery, such as when you have PRK

It's an expensive treatment, even if you have insurance

A small percentage of patients suffer from minor side effects, for example, halos during the night, or dry eyes that are frequent

The procedures may not be entirely covered by insurance. The patients who opt to undergo surgery may need more adjustments in the future, when there is a change to their eyes. This procedure is usually not advised for patients older than 40 because of other possible issues with vision that come from aging like presbyopia. The rule is that you should possess a stable prescription at least a year prior to surgery.

Some people are not a perfect person for undergoing the procedure, meaning people who do not have the choice of wearing eyeglasses or contacts. If you're suffering from a severe level of myopia, you could be an unsuitable patient for the procedure. Along with being costly the procedure is prone to risks as well as a variety of adverse effects.

The biggest issue is the well-known side-effect of dry eyes. Although it isn't likely to significantly alter your quality of life but it's something to take into consideration.

Chapter 4: Do You Really Require Glasses?

Much like many of you I was a beginner to using eyeglasses for a few years. Then, I decided to go for a simpler solution. I was in search of contacts. I prefer not wearing spectacles in all sorts of situations including sporting events. Contact lenses provided me with what spectacles could never do- the capability to look as though I were wearing normal glasses, without having a frame which there would be a blurred border. In the past I was able to use this method successfully and I was satisfied to discover a superior option than glasses. It was a great idea, I think.

There was only one issue with the price. The lenses were expensive. Because I was not a fan of washing lenses each evening, I went for those disposable ones that were available on a daily basis. In addition, I wasn't willing to run the risk of developing a serious eye infection if I failed to clean my lenses correctly. I wanted the absolute simplicity.

I was long-ago accustomed that wearing contact lens would become a fact throughout my life. After hearing about my close family and friends about their success with laser surgery I was pondering what it would be worth for me to shell out thousands of dollars for laser eye procedure. Should I keep using contact lenses? After doing the maths I thought it was an excellent deal to get laser surgery, compared to the thousands I'd invest in contacts.

Therefore, I set out to set up a consult regarding the procedure. Though the idea of spending this much money wasn't something I had a desire to do however, it was at least going to cost me nothing in order to get my good sight.

What is it going to set me back?

I was weighed down each year, of buying contacts. In the average, my dependence on AquaComfort Plus cost me close to 1,000 dollars each year. If you consider the 10 year expense, it could exceed the expense of procedure.

What a waste of time having to shell out thousands of dollars just to be able to look everyday? Normal vision sufferers have no idea of how fortunate they are not having to endure the stress of eye examinations and costly contact lenses.

Then, I became tired of spending so much that I began looking for ways to reduce the amount I spent on lenses. I initially tried purchasing lenses through 1-800-Contacts. Then, I went to Costco because they were in a position to offer a fantastic cost. I could save some money when compared to purchasing them from my optometrists. The only downside was when purchasing these online. This meant I would have be a struggle trying to pay for the purchase using the insurance for my eyes.

If you've ever attempted to make a claim via the insurance company of either of these providers It is, in short almost impossible.

The process isn't easy. There's a good chance that you'll return to your optometrist's clinic in order to determine how to encode the cost to be used for medical billing.

The procedure is so complex by insurance billing that it appears like it was created to make it difficult for you to go back to your optometrists. If you don't, you'll have an uphill task trying to collect money from the insurance company.

Although I had paid for my vision insurance with my employer, it became a hassle to file claims for purchases made by these organizations. The problem was that I didn't code my claim in the correct way or I had to jump through a different hoops to climb over. I realized quickly that it was just a waste of the time and effort to search for an amount that could take many hours, only to be rejected eventually.

Two options were available to me. One option was to take my optometrist to the nearest location and purchase a year's worth of glasses from them. I could then submit the purchase to my insurance for vision and expect that I will receive $100. Alternately, I could go to an alternative provider that is less expensive and not worry the whole process of submitting expenses.

To save speed and ease I usually opt for the former. Given that my vision insurance company is completely unresponsive to claims for contacts bought at Costco and Costco, I am unable to know why I'm paying my insurance provider.

It's as if that the whole process of purchasing contact lenses was designed to be a hassle and costly. Wouldn't it be nice to not have the need for contacts?

The loss of lenses when surfing

In the last few months, I picked the sport of surfing which I'd attempted several times throughout time and decided to move up to an entry-level. This was an excellent excuse to get back at the beach. I was able to take in nature, observe different kinds of wildlife such as harbor seals and pelicans looking at their next food source as they gracefully circled me. Plus, I was able to get an excellent workout by paddle-boarding past breaking waves.

However, I wasn't able to do it with the same enthusiasm like I'd imagined. When I paddled out, and then taking a ride in, or sometimes getting overwhelmed by waves, I'd often break a contact lenses. It is something about the broken waves, sand seaweed and the sheer force of water that does not seem to be in harmony with wear of contact lenses on the sea.

It's possible to store a backup supply of contacts in the car in case I needed them for the return trip. However, if they were lost at sea and it became difficult to be able to discern my surroundings, as well as anticipate the next wave that I needed to take. The result was that surfing turned into a pastime which was unsuitable for me unless I went through the use of lasers for vision.

Have you ever observed anyone online and wearing glasses? I thought about it as a possibility. Although it may sound funny however, it's not feasible due to the danger that they could be lost in the sea. For one thing, I'd be required to get home safe which means dropping my glasses or contacts would not be an possibility. It was also at this moment in my life that I overheard my family member discussing reversing myopia engaging in a different form of internet surfing. Online reading.

Is it possible to reverse myopia? I've worn contacts and glasses for a long time, and I'm sure this wasn't a scam or miscommunication. Through the years I've gained an increasing awareness of numerous misinformation on the internet. I was extremely skeptical and instantly dismissed the notion since I didn't think the possibility of it even being possible.

I was thinking it was a comedy. I thought, how did I not know about this before? I was wondering, how can it be treated? Why is it the first time that I'm being told about it at the age of my 30s?

I'd heard of eye exercises a few years ago, and concluded they are a complete unnecessary expense since they were not able to increase eyesight in a significant or quantifiable method. If they actually did improve eyesight the trick, they would surely have made it into journals of science and on medical websites.

Was this friend of mine, if any, talking about? They'd stumbled upon several YouTube videos as well as some internet communities where members had been discussing different methods for changing their vision.

The experience of surfing was the catalyst for me to take the decision to go through surgical vision correction using lasers. I decided that, as I planned to perform the procedure regardless, I'd consider being more open in regards to this potential reversal of myopia. Could it be feasible?

I made the decision then I was going to research about everything I could discover on the process of reversing myopia. I'd keep an open to the possibility, and make the fullest effort and try to determine whether I can achieve the same success as others were experiencing. What else was I going to gain, other than an additional contact lens in the Pacific Ocean?

If it did work this meant I would not have to spend thousands of dollars on surgery. The fact that I would never have to wear contacts or glasses never again, was an enormous incentive to give the procedure a try. I set out to do my own research into ways to repair the damage that I'd done to my vision in 20 years.

An opportunity to reveal

Armed by a mouse and a keyboard I started doing some studies. I started looking online. I researched accounts of different culture, like people who spend the majority of their time outdoors. The people in those cultures did not appear to be in a classroom with a Western-style environment. Nearly none of those living in these societies required vision correction. This is unusual since it's the complete opposite to what the majority of people across the globe does. Students enter an educational setting in their early years and then eventually require correction of vision. It was at this point that the association with eyeglasses and classrooms began to resemble more than a mere coincidence.

It was a long time before I could find some successful stories. There was an abundance of false information to sort through. Numerous articles advocated old-fashioned exercises for the eyes. It was evident that many of these techniques had no evidence of their effectiveness, success or even scientific backing.

The majority of the evidence I found didn't suggest any remedies that are natural however, I noticed there was a large quantity of proof. The data is what we'll examine in the next section provided evidence in favor to move away from using corrective lenses.

A few of the most prominent and reliable evidence of myopia reverse could be found in online forums. But, I'm still doubtful. Everyone can write wild tales of success. What makes these stories trustworthy?

I came across some anecdotal proof that people were able to recover their vision. However, I wasn't sure. There was no guarantee of success. who claim to have made huge advancement were not consistent. The degree of success varied. achievement. Some cases had there was no result was achieved.

I required more evidence prior to committing what appeared to be a massive amount of time needed for permanent improvement. I wanted to discover the most reliable evidence supported by science, not just any stranger on the internet.

I reflected on my youth and remembered that two of my relatives had been prescribed eyeglasses during their teenage years as I was. They both had mild myopia, and may not believe they had a need glasses. However They both utterly did not want to wear them. Perhaps they weren't looking very stylish in the clothes.

Today, many years later the pair of them have no glasses, however they can clearly see. How did they manage to avoid many years of wearing glasses when I was required to wear them for over two years? It could be that they accidentally applied one of the methods described in the book later on which helped them avoid aggravating their vision.

The experience was enough to have myself thinking about the possibilities of it succeeding. This encouraged me to make the attempt to improve my sight a serious attempt. I put off my plan to undergo the procedure and began the process of restoring my vision naturally. I didn't know what time it would be, but at the minimum,

I had evidence to prove it was possible. In the course of a few months, I've not just had the ability to quit relying on my contacts however, I also reached the point that I did not require any correction lenses in order to be able to see.

Chapter 5: Finding The Solution

Prior to beginning the journey to improve my vision, I was extremely doubtful. It is likely that you are uncertain about the likelihood of having a clearer vision again. If improving your vision is a possibility then why shouldn't everyone be aware of it? Everyone from athletes, doctors, scholar, pilot and celebrities will benefit from this understanding.

To determine the truth I read a lot of websites and forums where people were claiming to have seen a difference. There were scientific studies which provided me with proof that this could happen. I was concerned that I could spend my time doing nothing unless I had all the information. I required reliable research prior to being able to know that this was going to work.

The search for evidence

Do you think that myopia is prevalent within our society? Myopia's prevalence worldwide is at present hovering around 33%, and it is predicted to rise to 40% by 2030. 2 Billions suffer from the condition and the number will increase to millions within the next decade.

As I started to studies, I was astonished by a few aspects. The first was that I didn't think about how widespread the condition is throughout the globe. In addition, I did not comprehend why this condition is thought to be normal or even be considered something is not something we can control. Doesn't this seem like a very important issue the entire globe is confronting? Do we not need to pay more time to solve this issue, particularly when it affects so many of us?

The majority of people are quite content with having the expense of spending so much to have a clear view of the world. It's surprising to find to find that the focus isn't on the prevention of. In the meantime, generations of people are destined to live the cost that requires corrective lenses for a long time.

I could no longer live about this notion. I was fortunate to discover certain promising strategies to stop and treat myopia. I'm saying lucky since it was quite difficult to gather enough data for me to say that there's alternative options to treat myopia.

One of the most definitive evidences I have found was a research carried out on human people. The majority of them were predisposed to myopia while the remaining half did not have refractive errors. Results of this study was published as Human optical axial length as well as defocus, revealed that there was an evident variation in the length the eyes after applying an +3.0 diopter, or -3.0 diopter defocus on people in the study for a specified duration. Furthermore, the magnitude that changed was the same for those with myopia and those who did not have myopia.

In just one hour of focus the length of the eye was reduced by 10 millimeters. In comparison to the length of the human hair (between 17mm-181 millimeters) it is an extremely small difference in the length. But, if an eye is attracted to alter its length for such a brief duration What are the limitations of this transformation in the event that the same level of defocus remained for days, hours or even for weeks?

There is evidence to suggest that defocus actually increases the eyes and triggers it to become in length or width. The medical field does not know the reason or what causes this to happen in a biological sense However, it is something that is the focus of future studies.

Following the review of this study and analyzing it, I became more confident that there might be a straightforward solution for my problem with vision. I was impressed the possibility of the real possibility of reverse myopia.

The most important thing I learned from this research was the require to make conditions where my eyes suffer substantial blur or loss of focus.

I was pondering what I could do to reduce the size of my eyes? If I could maintain a steady defocus for several weeks, could I get rid of contacts and eventually be free of using contact lenses?

Another fascinating study was conducted with twin teens. The perfect situation where you are able to compare the experiences of two identical people with identical levels of myopia. The research tracked the growth of myopia in twins, known as twins A as well as Twin B. The two were both given contact lenses with a -1.75 diopter. The difference was that Twin A was assigned a bifocal lens with an +2.0 section that was part of the lens. Twin B received single-vision lenses.

In the course of an entire year Twin B's myopia increased by just 1.0 diopter. In contrast, Twin A showed almost none of the myopia progression at the rate of 0.13 diopter difference. After year two, Twin B was switched into the bifocal variation which showed myopia progress in the range of -0.28 diopter.

What we have learned from this research is the use of bifocal or additional lenses could be beneficial in the prevention of myopia. The study examined the outcomes of using a bifocal lens and stopped the progression of myopia. It is impossible to know how the outcome could look If Twin B wore +2.0 diopter lens, instead of Bifocal.

Alongside these informative research, I also went an additional study which revealed a lower prevalence of myopia in those who were more active outdoors. The main explanation is those who spent longer in bright, outdoors environments were more likely to take part in activities, such as athletics, which required the using distance vision, in contrast to indoor pursuits like reading.

Three conclusions are drawn from research for reversing myopia

In reviewing a number of studies about myopia-related research, I came to the conclusion that there are three primary conclusions that can be used in reversing myopia.

1. Do not use minus lenses unless required for a short duration

The first is to restrict your wearing of the minus glasses. Don't wear them unless you have to wear them wear them for short amounts for instance, while driving. At first, it is difficult to complete things such as work with the glasses. But, it is possible moving closer to what you're working on or opt for a less prescribed prescription, while working to improve the distance vision.

2. Develop good eyesight habits in particular when doing close tasks.

The other important aspect is to be aware of good vision behaviors. It is important to ensure that you are in a bright and well lit area if you're in the in the indoors. Be aware this: one of the major factors that cause myopia is an excessive amount of work near. If you are required to complete this type of job, you should remain as far from the work as possible.

Darkly lit areas make it harder to see clearly from an extended distance. One way to improve your vision is introduce more light that is preferably natural sunlight.

If you're reading the text, you should see an equilateral blur. If not, you're too close to the material you are reading or your computer screen. A slight blur can produce the same result similar to the study that we discussed earlier, that eyes can shrink in size when it's in an area with a significant amount of defocus. This will stimulate the eye to be able to perceive more clearly. The issue when reading text that's too crystal clear is that it forces your eyes to be inactive. If you're studying text close-up you are already in focus. Therefore, there's nothing to do so there's no incentive that can stimulate your eyes to work better.

3. Wear reading glasses while performing in the vicinity of work

Thirdly, reading glasses should be worn if you are unable to physically stand or sit far enough to perform close work. They can cause some blurring while working in close distances. As an example, when using smartphones, the majority of users are using it less than an elbow's distance or when using corrective lenses. In these close proximity you should wear lenses for reading as text is usually very clear. It will also allow us to maintain a the defocus of the material we read. You will notice that reading glasses are the best tool you can employ to battle myopia as they can cause blurring.

We have now observed that numerous research studies have pointed to the advantages of diopter lenses with plus. They can either eliminate or decrease myopia. The conclusion is the reading glasses or even more lenses will prove helpful in increasing your vision naturally.

Chapter 6: A Dramatic Improvements

In the event that the COVID-19 outbreak which was supposed to be a threat in 2020 in 2020, I'm not certain that I would have even had the opportunity to improve my eyesight. It is likely that I would be unable to locate an efficient way to get to work since I'd have to wear contacts throughout all entire day. The likelihood is that I'd already gone through laser surgery and gone forward with my daily life. In the midst of the pandemic, there was a lot of anxiety and doubt. This was an extremely strange moment, especially during March, a time when people were convinced that closing offices, schools, as well as many other businesses, would be for a short period of time or even just a few months. It's all we have seen how this came out.

I was fortunate enough at the time that I had an employment. It was more fortunate to find a job that permitted me to work remotely. In the event that offices closed, I was allowed to work at home for the remainder all year. Because I'd conducted quite a lot of studies into ways to overcome myopia, I was able to have an almost limitless amount of time to study ways of improving my eyesight from the comfort of at home. In the end, I realized I was in the right place at the time, and it was very good for me.

My initial point is: legally blind

As I was first beginning to wear glasses when I was in my teen years I was given a range of between -2.0 or -3.0 diopter lenses to each eye. As a result of my worsening myopia due to constant wear during the subsequent years, my glasses prescription became higher and stabilized at -4.0 in both eyes. It continued to be that way for more than 10 years after. It was at this moment when I started working on the distance of my vision.

If I had not worn corrective lenses, then I might incapable of even being capable of reading the 20/200 line of the eye chart. Did you be aware that if a person cannot discern the letter that is the largest in this chart, then you're legally blind?

My main goal was to restore the vision clarity I experienced as a youngster. I wanted to have 20/20 vision without the need for the need for corrective lenses. I wasn't sure of the time frame it would take to achieve this, however I knew that I would need an easy way of tracking my progress throughout the months and weeks which followed.

What can I do to ensure I could track the progress I made in a reproducible method? The majority of individuals have difficulty focusing even in dim lighting and particularly in the evening. This was the reason I looked at the tools used by optometrists in their practice eye charts. I found an online version which I set in my bedroom which could also be used for an office. The space had a lot of lighting from the windows. The setup was perfect as it let me check my vision in similar conditions by using an ordinary chart.

Weekly updates

When I measured my improvements each week I was in understanding the changes happening to my vision, and the speed at which my vision was getting better. I was unable to discover any similar logs online, which is why I thought of creating my own log to make a reference.

I've broken down my progress every couple of weeks. This is a disclaimer. This was an opportunity for me to keep track of how fast I could work through the process of removing corrective lenses and still be able to complete routine tasks, and read from a reasonable distance. This does not mean I was able to see 20/20 when switching to a lower power lens. But, it could provide a direction to those who require an approximate time frame to use on your way toward good vision.

The improvement did not come anytime soon than at minimum every two or three weeks. Apart from the techniques discussed in the later parts of the book The main strategy I utilized throughout my entire time was to decrease the diopter strength required for clarity as fast as I could. Once I was used to a certain amount of power then I made myself switch to a lower power lens.

It meant I'd have ordered slightly weaker contact lenses. I ordered -3.0, -2.0, and -1.0 together with an additional couple of +1.0 reading glasses. The goal was to be able to read and focus at a an appropriate distance, because my vision had improved over the months.

When it comes to a routine, I needed to be working. My desk job is a standard job and I have to be able to read from a reasonable distance this is the reason I couldn't just quit wearing contacts. When I started my process, wearing only my eyes alone, I could discern or read clearly from the maximum distance of 25 cm and that was just the right amount blur to me at the time. If you're fortunate enough not to have such a high amount of myopia like I did, it is recommended that you be sure to stop using lenses with minus totally and relocate towards a point away from your job where you're in a position to read around the blur mark.

Think about how little of the distance can be. It's not practical sitting that near a screen for a computer. If you're beginning with a blur level greater than 25cm then you might find it relaxing to be at a desk while working. If not, you'll have be creative in increasing the distance to the monitor or use gradually less the strength of lenses, as I used to do.

Even though the prescription I was wearing was -4.0 diopters, in order to bring the defocus I needed to my routine, I was looking to get -3.0 diopters. To reach this point I put on +1.0 diopter glasses for reading when I wore -4.0 contacts. The primary reason I used just one diopter reduction was the fact that I was finding it difficult sitting at a distance from the computer's screen in order to read emails and complete daily chores. But, using gradually less abrasive lenses over the course of a few months I was able gradually ease myself from the use of any lens that was minus work.

I used this pair for between 8 and 9 hours for work. I did not wear glasses for the remainder of the time. At times, I would wear contact lenses for about thirty minutes, if I needed to go someplace.

Here is the record I used to keep track of the contact lens strength I was using and how long in addition to wearing +1 reading glasses. Once I was able moving from -3 lenses or -2 lens, usually I did not need to wear reading glasses during the initial week or two since my eyes were continuing to adapt to the lower intensity. Then, I'd begin wearing the +1 lens with -2 contacts, and continue for several weeks until I didn't need contact lenses in the first place.

Week Contact lens Corrective by +1.0 reading glasses

1-3 -4.0 -4.0 to -3.0

4-6 -3.0 -3.0 to -2.0

7-9 -2.0 -2.0 to -1.0

10-11 -1.0 -1.0 to 0

12-13 -1.0 0

14-beyond 0 +1.0

In the beginning I was wearing +1.0 reading glasses because I didn't know what capabilities I'd ultimately require to build. In conjunction with contacts this allowed me to keep a certain distance from the screen of my laptop so that I could retain a blurred image that I found helpful for encouraging my eyes to concentrate and eliminate the blur. This is the main reason in my ability to see such rapid improvements in myopia reduction. It was difficult to constantly work with blurry images, but I'm convinced that this was the most important reason for my growth.

The weekly charts show what lenses I wore during this particular phase of my procedure. I usually started out with a less powerful contact lens. However, as my eyes improved in the subsequent months, I was able to begin wearing reading glasses on top of my contacts in order to create a small difficulty. The practice of wearing them for a long time each day was highly efficient. In fact, it was so efficient that, when I conducted my next eye exam I discovered that I could better read the smaller fonts in the chart of my eyes.

Through these two weeks, I observed how my point of blur has altered. In this case, the reason for blur refers to the distance between your eyes to standard text, such as 12 point font. When I first began trying to make improvements, this distance was about 25cm. In the following weeks and onwards, the distance increased until it was 35 50, 40 and then 60+cm. I decided not to keep any logs of the distance blurred as there was too much variation in a week-to-week basis which made it difficult to determine the exact distance.

It's crucial to understand that although I could use gradually weaker lenses each few weeks, it doesn't mean my vision had improved to an equal reading in an eye examination. It did however fulfill my initial purpose of not wearing any glasses for my everyday tasks.

In the course of a couple of months after a few months, I was able to totally stop wearing contact lenses. But, I did regularly wear my reading glasses to work throughout my day, as I discovered they were helpful in enhancing my vision distance.

What time did it require me to restore my sight?

I stopped wearing the minus lenses after around three months. this was perfectly fine as I was able to work from outdoors or at home without having to be able to see with laser-like vision. In the end, it took around nine months until I was frequently looking at the 20/20 line on an eye chart.

It is my opinion that the majority of my rapid improvement occurred during the initial three months. I did experience slow progress throughout the remainder of the period. It could be due to my years of wearing contact lenses every day that my eyes were unnaturally forced to an extent that the ciliary muscles were overloaded? Could that be the reason it took an extremely quick procedure to allow that muscle back to its original activity? Maybe.

I didn't know the length of time it would last, but I would've been beneficial to be aware of this prior to paying more for the additional contact lenses of different strength that I bought at the time, but didn't ever need.

In the beginning of the procedure, I had no idea of how long the process would take, or the extent it could be successful. When I finally crossed the point, I was thrilled. When I regained the clarity of vision I only imagine being able to see as a kid and I realized I'd saved myself from the years of spending cash and time, as well as frustration and effort on purchasing contact lenses, and also avoiding the laser procedure. In the meantime I was a bit confused about how many people do not know about the methods to reverse myopia? Is it not widely recognized that all you need is to know a couple of tricks to correct myopia?

Since the majority of strategies I tried was based on trials and errors, I experienced some difficulty in my ability discern the 20/20 line. I'm confident of the fact that I would have achieved faster gains than the nine month experience I had. Through experimenting with different methods that I found to be not as effective, it's evident that the best approach will result faster advancement. If you're like me, that you are able to take shortcuts using only the most efficient methods in order to restore the natural sight as fast as you can.

In the past, I'd made significant progress over the past couple of weeks, I became more comfortable in working using the same techniques I'd used previously. Being not able to discern using entirety diopter of lower lenses confirmed that this method could be effective.

After three months, my eyesight would change from being unable to read more than 25 centimeters from my eye, to being able read easily at a distance of over a meters away. I had made such a leap that I could no longer feel comfortable needing any correction lenses when driving during the day. However, I was still not able to be able to drive in the evening and so I opted for -1.0 and -2.0 contacts for those times when I needed them. When I was driving during the day, I was able to verify that I was able to discern the 20/40 lines, that is the legal standard across the world and is required in many places in the area where I reside.

Discovering ways to boost vision with trial and trial and

Two of them were factors that contributed to improving. One of them was keeping the best eye habits and wearing reading glasses whenever feasible to be able to read text that is blurred. Second, go out. It seems like a simple task isn't it? Going outside is a crucial part of the procedure. While inside it isn't a great chances for you to let your eyes to view objects from afar. When I say distance, I'm talking about anything that is six metres (20 feet) far away. It is achievable as soon as you take a step out. While outdoors, your eyes will have an opportunity to look at the vast majority of far-off and moving things. Things with high contrast like the edge of buildings, branches of trees, as well as power lines are great for watching. All of these are great things that you can try to concentrate on and observe easily. Do your best to constantly bring distant things into your sharp focus.

The view is better when it is a bright, clear day. It is likely that it isn't possible to see the same when it's cloudy. Also, get out and go for a walk and leave your home frequently. If you don't, your travels is going to be a lot slower.

The reasons why others might not have been able to find their sense of vision

I've heard of numerous people who failed using the same methods I took I am sceptical that there might not have been a complete commitment to the limitation of use of minus lenses. Stop using corrective lenses as a substitute and stop making them a means to get around. From my experiences, reading emails or other messages in a blurry manner is essential to make progress. It is important to not do these things, or you can slow down the pace of your learning.

Don't spend enough time each day with reading glasses

We will be reverting to corrective lenses as it's simpler to carry out every day routine

Recognizing that it takes commitment on a daily basis for months in order in order to make improvement

Reading from a distance that is large enough that it creates a sufficiently strong blur

Chapter 7: Manage Your Expectations

Today, users have learned to anticipate instant feedback in all areas of life. Take a look at the various social media applications which you use on a daily basis. Most of them have been specifically designed to notify you or send notifications when someone else is a fan of your content, leaves comments, or even communicates with you directly.

The way you shop has altered in recent times. Before, you'd go to the store for a drive-through to an electronic retailer, purchase a cable to hook your brand new television to two speakers, then return to your to your home, only to be shocked when you realized it was 2 inches too short. In the end, you'd need to repeat the drive to obtain the proper size of the cable. Today, you will be able to get the cable tomorrow not even leaving your home.

We have become so used to immediate gratification that doing long or difficult tasks are far out of our thoughts. The majority of people prefer to take the elevator instead of taking the stairs. It's faster and comfortable.

For improving vision, the notion of instantaneous gratification doesn't exist. It is therefore essential to have reasonable expectations about how fast and how long it is expected to be achieved.

If you had promised to never wearing corrective lenses since today I'm sure that your eyesight will eventually be restored to normal. It's likely to be a few years before you could implement the strategies described in later chapters.

It might be beneficial should you misplace your glasses, and found yourself on an island that was deserted with plenty of food and other necessities to survive. In the end, at this moment, all that you're left with is the clock. You'll have plenty of time to regain your vision and then have the ability to share with anyone else about the miraculous transformation.

In the beginning, it is important be able to set the right expectations and ensure that we're not chasing miraculous results when we ought to concentrate on small victories that can provide you with confidence in the fact that you're progressing towards having a clearer vision. As an example, having clear vision and having 20/20 vision can be assessed at various points in the process, in several stages.

Stage 1. Clear vision -3.0 diopter correctional lenses

Stage 2. Clear vision utilizing -1.0 diopter correctional lenses

Stage 3. Clear vision with no any correctional lenses

We are unable to determine the amount of time between milestones simply since there's no huge collection of patients who have recorded their improvement in vision. My personal improvement as a benchmark but there are far numerous variables that make it difficult for me to state with certainty that you've progressed from -3.0 up to -2.0 lenses within three months. It is possible that you are with an overcorrection, or you might not be able to keep up your pace on weekends and this could slow your progress.

Which is the best place to start?

If you've just begun using corrective lenses or if you are suffering from very slight myopia, you're extremely blessed to have discovered this guide. The chances are that you'll have the ability to restore your clarity much quicker than the rest of us. Not only will you be able stop the further decline, but quicker restore the damage that has been done to your distant vision. If you're like the majority of us the recovery process will be significantly longer.

There's a possibility that you might have undercorrected vision. Are you able to read lower letters of the 20/20 line of the standard eye chart for example, that 20/13 line? If yes, then you may possess more powerful lenses than what that you truly require. In contrast If you find it difficult to see 20/20 lines even with the current lenses you have You could be suffering from undercorrected vision.

If your initial point of departure is similar or better than the point at which I started (I had -4.0 lenses) The amount of time required to return to clear, normal vision is at a minimum, which can be as long as several months. How fast you progress will depend on the amount of time dedicated to the strategies discussed further in the book.

In an age that is populated by people who are used to expecting things to occur immediately, the road toward improvement in your vision can be unexpectedly slow. It requires a lot of dedication and a lot of time each day to make sure you are making significant advancement. Prior to starting with this, it's important consider whether you're willing to invest an investment that is so significant in time.

It is not a problem having a desire not to invest an enormous amount of time and energy in this endeavor even though there are a variety of "quick fixes" such as using your current corrective lenses, or even pursuing surgical procedures using lasers. If you're taking this course, it is likely that you're not among those who have any desire to try the techniques described here.

When you think about it this way the speed at which improvement occurs depends on you. What amount of time per day are you able to dedicate to enhancing your eyesight? It's entirely in your hands.

There are those who devote a lot of time and even the whole day adhering the plan, and other people will struggle only for just a few hours every day since they can't invest more. What ever your preference might be, remember that the pace of progress will slow in the shorter time you dedicate to the task.

How long does this process take?

Although there are far too many variables to offer an exact timeframe however, I'd suggest that the minimum of 3 months. Since we don't know if you have myopia that is near two digits, or if it is mild and mild, it's impossible to suggest a specific time frame. I'm able to tell you the time it took me to get my vision back and also how fast it may help you.

Chapter 8: There Are No Tools That You Require Are The Tools You

I'm happy to announce that I've got good news as well as I've got negative good news and bad. The good news is that there are just two things will be required on the road to correct your myopia The other one can be found for free.

The very first chart you will easily locate online. Simply open your preferred search engine and enter "Snellen chart."

There are plenty of free examples, but you should try to find one designed specifically to be used at the distance of 6 meters, or 20 feet. There is charts designed to be used at 10 feet but bear your eyes on the 20 foot version as it might be less accurate in comparison to the 20-foot version. The reason 20-foot versions are the best choice is because it accurately depicts viewing from a distance reality-based perspective than the 10-foot version. Get a good Snellen chart, or create one online. It is an essential device that can allow you to monitor your progress in the coming months and weeks.

Another eye chart, called"the logmar chart. It is typically used in professional settings as opposed to the more traditional Snellen chart. The Snellen chart is the one that most people have come across. It's easy to comprehend and operate.

However, the downside is that you'll have to shell out some cash for a few pair of reading glasses or even more lenses. They are generally priced with prices less than $10 and can be purchased from every grocery store, drugstore and even online. It's great that they're not expensive as you'll require a range of capabilities throughout the course of.

Even though you'll struggle at first when you begin in focusing on anything using lenses that are stronger but you'll eventually require between +1 and +6, contingent upon how fast you are used to them close work. The quicker you work toward being able make use of the larger lenses on a regular basis as well, the quicker your vision for distance will improve. Stronger reading glasses are more beneficial to you as your sight grows. If you see a plateau in your improvement after using the +3 lens, for instance this is an signal that it is time to change to the larger lens so that you can continue to progress toward 20/20 and better vision.

In accordance with how serious your current myopia may be it is possible to buy gradually weaker lenses or contact. If, for instance, you currently wear -6.0 lenses or contacts but you are using -6.0 glasses, you won't be able to perceive everything through the lens. All will appear blurred.

Most of the time, you won't have to begin using reading glasses until approximately the diopter level of corrective needed to have clarity of vision. Simply remove your spectacles and you will have enough to allow your eyes to grow longer. It may be difficult to perform certain tasks throughout your day without having enough correction. If you are looking to achieve most rapid results then you must get rid of your lenses that are minus and make a concerted effort to use increasingly more powerful reading glasses.

In order to help you progress In the beginning, particularly it is possible that you will require assistance from an optometrist. Since I was using gradually less abrasive contact lenses in the initial few months it is possible this to be the best way to go about the improvement of your own.

The research suggests the need to avoid any unnecessary use of prescription lenses with minus ones but it could be quite difficult working when you can't discern clearly beyond a specific distance. In such a case it makes more sense to choose a less restrictive prescription so that you can stand and work from an appropriate distance.

In time, you'll eventually become able to be able to work with them. Of course, you will need be able to change your distance to what you're working but you'll have no need for the minus lens and will be able to begin by using the plus lens, starting with the one that is plus as you become more familiar with stronger lenses.

The more time you'll spend with plus lenses and the sooner you start wearing stronger and more powerful as well as lenses that are suitable for work in close proximity as well as the more quickly you'll be able to attain 2020 vision.

To improve your eyesight, you'll need to choose the opposite lens to the one recommended through your optometrist. It's not as obvious adding lenses to your vision can allow users to eliminate the lenses that are minus.

As a conclusion this is the sole requirements you'll require in order to bring back your sight. How much do the lenses or glasses costs you each year? Consider the amount of time and energy required going to annual exam? It's a lot of effort to keep an up-to-date prescription only to order the same contact lenses or glasses when your prescription hasn't changed throughout the several years. Wouldn't it be nice to have return your money and time?

I was able to purchase reduced force contacts to aid in my process of improvement. However, this is a costly method of achieving the goal. If this is a good fit to you, attempt to use similar steps. An alternative that is more economical is to purchase more powerful reading glasses, which gradually decrease your prescription when wearing the prescription you already have.

The best part about this approach is that it's extremely affordable compared to the amount you have to pay to get your vision solutions. You only need to be diligent every day to make sure you succeed. If you are using more than four types of lenses, they're affordable that you should not need to pay over $50 in order to restore your vision back to 20/20. If you do your research and compare prices, you might get less than that.

We'll now dive into how you can use these tools to help comprehend why they are effective. We'll start with the chart of Snellen.

First Tool A Snellen eye chart

What do you mean by an Snellen chart?

The Snellen chart refers to an eye which is utilized to gauge the visual acuity or the clarity of your sight. The chart has many rows of letters which gradually shrink in size as you progress further down the chart.

The Snellen chart is one of the most commonly used eye chart to measure an individual's eye's visual ability. It's an eye test that was first introduced in 1862. The chart is set in a space of 20 feet, which is about 6 meters. The person is required to gaze at the chart and then read any line that they're in a position to read from that distance. Thus, anyone who has normal vision will be able to discern line 8 of the chart. This is equivalent to 20/20 vision.

Let's look at what this number signifies. The first "20" indicates how many feet away the chart is located, while the number 2 indicates how far a person with normal vision will be able to discern the identical line. For instance that a person only capable of reading line 6 (or the 20/40 line) can only see clearly from 20 feet, the distance a person who has normal vision could see at 40 feet.

When you begin the journey towards improving your vision it is possible that you are unable to discern between the lines 20/100. It's fine. your progress through the techniques described in this article will allow your eyes to slowly improve until they are able to see 20/20 lines or even better.

There are numerous online sources for printing or downloading an Snellen chart free of charge. Important to know whether the chart is located at the 10th or 20th feet. Choose one that shows the length from the top in the diagram. If you don't have room at home It is fine to go with the version that measures 10 feet. But, it is important to know that this version can not exactly replicate the efficiency of the 20-foot version. It is possible to look at the 20/50 line in the 10 foot chart, however there is a good chance that it is not possible to read that same line on this 20-foot version. Remember this while you're evaluating your improvement.

If you'd like an elegant and professional-looking one You can locate some to purchase from these links.

The best-selling eye chart to usage at 20 feet.

Popular eye chart for use at 10 feet

A proper placement is required to guarantee consistent result.

If you've located an area of your house in which you can put the chart in make sure that the area is lit properly. It is recommended to use sunlight, but it isn't consistent through the day and this isn't the best option. Unprofessional lighting results in irregular and unsatisfactory results, which I've found extremely frustrating. Use the desk lamp directed at the chart or like it, which can provide reliable results. It is possible to get more precise results, and possibly more rapid progress when the chart is properly illuminated, at least by similar type and amount of illumination.

Are you able to convert the Snellen readings to a comparable prescription?

In short, no precisely. Some of you may wonder whether there's a method to translate the results taken from the Snellen chart to the kind of prescription you'll need. There is no way to change Snellen readings into diopter correction. It is impossible to get zero because it implies you're in vision over an endless distance. 20/20 does not really represent zero. It's technically -1.0 If you consider calculations to determine the conversion. Also, it is you can see clearly of 1 millimeter (about three feet) that is the equivalent of the standard for normal vision.

An actual illustration of this is the time I embarked on my myopia-reversal journey. I was prescriber-4.0 for some time. This is which is 20/80 or 0.25 millimeters. But, when I tried it I couldn't discern the 20/80 line in any way. That's why it's impossible to make the conversion between these two levels. But it can be beneficial to take the information below for reference.

Snellen

chart reading Maximum clear vision distance Diopter correction required

20/80 25cm -4.00

20/40 50cm -2.00

20/20 100cm -1.00

Actual corrections are established by an eye specialist or by the trial-and-error method with a lens that has an exact power and observing your own eye acuity using the Snellen chart (for instance, you can wear -1.0 lens, and test how well you read a 20/20 lines).

As per the conversion those who has 20/20 vision may discern better than a clear image in 1 one meter. But, it isn't the most accurate way to convert since those who has 20/20 vision is able to discern clearly even greater than 1 millimeter. However, it is important to think about the conversion to figure out what corrections an optometrist could offer depending on the distance you be able to see.

The lighting is essential to get exact readings

Once you've got the Snellen chart setup it will allow you monitor your progress by being in a place that is consistent within the home where you can check your vision in the same lighting conditions.

We'll take a closer look at the second tool you'll use to aid in improving your vision: the reading glasses, also known as additional lenses.

2. Reading glasses beginning with +1.0

Reading glasses are offered in various qualities and can be purchased buy without a prescription. Another benefit is that they're extremely affordable. There is no worry about them falling off or harming the lenses like you do with prescription glasses. Reading glasses are able to make everything you look at. Additionally, in terms of improving vision They allow users to add a small focus on the text you're reading.

In the event that you are going to be using glasses for reading, you could need to own several pairs. The lens of +1.0 could be suitable to use your computer, however it is possible that you require +2.0 when you're using your phone, or reading from a distance that is closer to the computer. In the following section we'll take an in-depth look at how make use of these lenses in order to improve your eyesight to see.

After extensive testing using reading glasses with varying powers, it's evident that many people are able to keep using more powerful lenses with increases by 1.0 diopter. This lets you continue pushing the eye to expand your distance until the point of blur.

My favorite reading classes can be found by clicking this link. It comes as a pack of six items, which means you will have a pair in your bag at all times and don't have to fret all that much about getting them damaged or lost. The price is very reasonable, and they appear great on females as well as males.

Traditional reading glasses in black

If you believe that you'll also require various lower strengths minus lenses in the beginning of your journey to improvement and you'll find they may add significant on the price, but it could also be a necessity problem in the way toward clearer vision. If your vision is -3.0 or more it is possible that you will struggle in your daily activities and even work with a no-reduced prescription for minus. But, if you're close to -2.0 or greater it is likely that you will remove your lens minus immediately and start using the additional lenses.

Optometrists tend to be open to prescribing less strength, if you make a request for the reduction. The reason could be such as:

I experience more strain in my eyes while wearing a higher prescription

I'd like stay clear of glasses for every day since I need glasses only to see for short periods of time

You would rather not be astonished by the intensity of correction because you don't see this as necessary to live a normal life

A simpler method I've discovered is to use something similar to the 800-contacts app. This will allow you to conduct your own test and allow you to find a weaker pair contacts.

If you're already a user of contact lenses and want to upgrade your contacts, it will help make life times simpler when you are striving to improve your performance quickly.

Chapter 9: What Can You Do To Increase Your Distance Vision

On a larger scale how to enhance distant vision would be to eliminate the lenses that are minus as soon as you can. The goal is to reduce gradually the power of the prescription lenses you already have gradually until you are able to complete most tasks near with naked eyes. Then, you'll gradually switch to more powerful plus lenses until you can achieve perfect vision in both distant and close distances.

A summary of the improvement in vision procedure

While you go through the book, and start to implement methods to improve your vision It might be beneficial to know the overall outline of the procedure since it offers a path starting from the beginning and ending at the conclusion.

1. Start point

a. If your prescription exceeds 2, decrease it by gradually weakening your lenses until you are able to reduce it to 2.

b. If your reading level is the level of -2 or lower, then you are able to start using +1.0 reading glasses right away until you are reading text that is blurred.

2. Continuous improvements

a. Improve until you don't need less lenses to work near.

b. Change to +2 and more powerful reading glasses until you can improve your natural distance vision

C. Continue to use progressively stronger reading glasses, particularly after you have reached a certain level.

3. Final point

a. If you're using from +4 to +6 reading glasses in close work, you'll have within 20/20 vision

b. It is only necessary to wear reading glasses if you can physically be seated far enough from the work area, and you don't require any kind of lenses at all.

Step 1: Restrict the your use of existing corrective lenses for short periods of time, when complete clarity is needed.

I'd like to make it so easy as saying you could just take off the glasses. Unfortunately, in the early stages of your journey, you'll be required to wear them for different things. As an example, you can't legally drive without having at least 20/40 vision, in many areas therefore, do not try to drive with out corrective lenses.

If you take off the glasses you wear and read the computer's screen or monitor it is likely that the display appears blurred when you are a specific distance. The distance you move is crucial to improving your vision.

Second step: read on the edges of blur

It is generally said that there are three places that text can be transparent, blurry or is impossible to read.

When you focus the majority of the time reading in the second position by reading at a second distance, your eyes are able to draw the text in focus. When you apply this to routine, you'll often notice that the text is almost completely transparent. For a brief moment. If you keep doing the daily routine, you'll be able to see improvement.

The distance that you are able to clearly read text is also increasing. In the example above I first began reading in the blurred area that I was unable to see clearly over 25 cm or more. In about 6-8 weeks I could read clearly at 30 cm, 35 cm and then 40 cm. Eventually, the text became blurred for me to see.

The reading glasses can be extremely beneficial for the development process. When you try to read a book is in your hand, based upon your visual acuity, it could become difficult for you to maintain the text at an appropriate distance that it blurs the text. Utilizing +1.0 Reading glasses you are able to raise the book up to a suitable reading distance and not stretch your arms to far. If you're in a workstation and are to read emails, it is best to set your seat and monitor in a position that will let you read in some blur. You should move your chair and screen towards the right distance so that you can ensure that you are reading in a blur.

Since this is the basis of the way you can trigger the eye to change to improve clarity. Below is another method of looking at text that is blurred from various distances with the +1 lenses.

One of the most effective methods for increasing the clarity of your vision

Image 1 is transparent and doesn't pose any obstacle for the eyes to discern any blue.

Image 2 is critical as it shows you where exactly the text should be. Choose a distance which allows you to maintain this significantly sharper blur. It is still possible to read the words but it does not give the user enough difficulty because it's not completely crystal clear. It's important to remain in this range, or perhaps a little sharper, since it is the way to achieve an improvement.

Image 3 appears to be extremely blurred, and is more or less difficult to comprehend. This happens because you move further away from text and doesn't assist the eye in staying focused. Thus, there's no requirement to keep in this position.

If you are reading at Image 2 distance, you continuously encourage your eye to concentrate upon the words. If you find reading the text to be difficult, you'll have to shift a more closer in order to be able to look at text that is slightly blurred. After a few hours of reading from this angle, you will be capable of "clear" the blurred text by weaving the text which was blurry before, and it now looks very clear when viewed through lenses. The clarity of the text will change over the period you're viewing it, but the more you're able to maintain blurred text, the greater improvement you'll see.

Through the course of several weeks, you'll notice an improvement in your eyes that allows you to go further and further away from text. This is the goal of this course: to slowly improve your eye's ability to focus on distance.

In the past you will recall that there are many ways to cause myopia, as well as the way it gets worse with time because of bad vision habits.

The quality of text is constantly changing when your eyes try to find the right focus. However, trying to view the text in a clear way at a distance 2. You are forcing your eyes to adjust. This is arguably the most important aspect of the process. In comparison to simply wearing reading glasses all entire day, I noticed that actively trying to eliminate blurred text produced quicker and noticeable effects.

Since my day-to-day activities involve reading lots of software agreements and agreements, I could complete the task for hours. I was always at a distance which blurred the text as illustrated on Image 2 and trying to erase the text that was blurred.

It is easier to achieve faster results If you're able to duplicate what I wrote and clearly blur the text for all day long as you are able to. You must ensure that you make time for breaks so that you don't exhaustion and strain.

Most people, particularly people who work at desks that don't read contract documents all time, the ideal method is to use this with your email, and any other devices you employ for work for example, internet browsers. It is likely that you may work more slowly than you would normally because you're struggling to read. But, you must persevere and know you'll see be benefited.

Step 3: Purchase an assortment of gradually less powerful lenses which allow readers to work near the edges of blur

The blurred eyes caused by the constant wear force the eye to adjust. Be aware that having corrective lenses on all day for a long time has led to the eye to increase in size. It was able to adapt then, and is likely to adapt as you make it be in a space that is blurrier, which can be caused when you are seated further away from the material you work with or by adding additional lenses. These studies show how a tiny duration of wear glasses helps the eye decrease in length, and brings your eye closer to attaining the natural clarity of vision.

The most effective method I've discovered is to utilize the latest technology for your benefit. Every business has a smartphone app nowadays. 1-800-Contacts is a mobile app that lets you renew your prescription for contact lenses by through their online eye examination according to the state in which you live in. I've discovered that it is easy to perform the eye examination several times, and receive lower strength prescriptions rapidly.

It is the most efficient method to obtain all your contacts that you require. This can be expensive but it's essential for you to gradually move away from the existing prescription, and eventually to having no prescription.

I'm currently unaware of any vendor who allows the purchase of contact lenses without having a legally valid prescription.

In addition, if you build an excellent relationship with your optometrist, they will be open to offering the patient a less expensive prescription for contact lenses, which will allow you to buy lenses from any retailer you prefer.

If you would prefer wearing glasses, there are handful of eyeglass manufacturers which cut out middlemen and deliver directly to the customer generally without the need to submit a copy of the prescription.

Eye Buy Direct is a highly recommended site that has cheap frames, as well as an extensive range of frames.

If you prefer, Zenni Optical is another high-rated provider that could let you purchase several pair of glasses with lower prescriptions as you progress through your progress.

Achieving the correct level of correction that is reduced will enable your progress to be faster which is why it's crucial for you to receive the correct prescription at a lower level as required.

Step 4: Take minimum 1-2 hours outdoors taking in the natural world, observing it from a position with plenty of sunlight.

Are you sure that humans developed the ability to stay in the dark for long hours every day? Absolutely it isn't. Our species has evolved to spend the majority of the day in the outdoors, hunting and gathering. In the last 200 or so years did humans have to be indoors for extended periods. In the past, human beings worked in fields, and tending cattle.

The earlier study in the book examined those who spent a specific portion of their lives outdoors and showed an elongated period of myopia for those who are more active outdoors. It's not a coincidence.

If you've ever bought an lightbulb from a retailer and noticed that they're available with different brightness levels. They're usually rated based on the amount of lumens that a lightbulb will produce. The more lumens is brighter, the more powerful the bulb and the more light it will emit.

In the same way, Lux is another measure of light that measures the amount of lumens contained within a square meters. If we look at the lights in outdoor and indoor environments It should come as not a surprise to see significant distinction. What is the extent of the distinction is there? Based on a study of myopia prevention the amount of light emitted in lux could be around 1,000 times greater than the indoor light. [6]

Did you try to wander around in the dark or even woken up at the end of the night, searching for something darkness? It is likely that you had difficulties seeing things because of the absence of light. Perhaps you utilized a flashlight to view more clearly.

In the same way, we could look at this as a contrast between outdoor and indoor lighting. Being outside is like switching on a light bulb everywhere and allows people to observe objects in stunning clarity.

So, it's vital to take all the time possible outdoors. You can aid your eyes to focus more effectively as everything are naturally clearer in the outdoors.

The study which examined the light levels was also able to determine that glasses allowed minimum 1700 lux of light to illuminate the eye outside as opposed to the normal indoor light which is around 125 lux.

Since sunglasses block away a significant amount of sunlight however, I don't recommend wearing them until you've made major advancements in reverseing myopia. One of the main reasons is the fact that you'll have an advantage in giving your eyes all the light they can each day. This helps in preventing and reversal, but also with the treatment of myopia.

5. Transition into using more powerful reading glasses

Once you've been capable of using progressive lenses with reduced minus and you'll no require all lenses to perform everyday tasks. Once that day is here you are awestruck! Then you can begin living your life without glasses, minus your vision when you are at your work!

In reality, you may never have 20/20 vision. If you want to work close there is a need the use of additional lenses. I discovered that the +1 lens worked well enough to see significant improvements. In the end, however, I came to the point where I realized I'd need more reading glasses. However, for me it was only by trials and errors to discover this was the next stage of making further improvements.

One important thing to remember in this regard is to make an effort to bring images to the center of your vision in particular when wearing reading glasses. If you are able to get your eyes to concentrate, and the longer your vision remains clear more rapid your progress will occur.

If you've made enough progress to utilize +1.0 lenses and are comfortable with them after some time then you should increase the intensity to +2.0 when you're at ease. This can help you maintain development of your eyesight. The more you are aggressively using more powerful Plus lenses, the more quickly you'll improve. I squandered a lot of time trying various techniques like using +1.0 contacts for months, and I discovered that none was as efficient than switching to larger plus lenses. The most powerful lenses I could look through and put in many hours a day was the best to improve my skills. This was similar to cracking the code, and eventually helped me make rapid progress while shifting between 20/30 and 20/20.

In the next part in the next section, we'll take a review of some great practices for vision and ways to incorporate them into your life for a better chance of improvement in the coming three or six months or as long as it takes in order to return to regular sight.

Clearing Blurred Text

It can be difficult and uncomfortable for a lot of individuals. The method involves focusing on objects with sufficient clarity like an eye chart from Snellen, which lets you attempt to remove small, blurred letters. If you are sitting on an eye chart at the proper distance it is possible that you will not be able read small rows of letters. But, you can go through the rows until reach one can be easily distinguished. Once you've found it then, focus on the row directly beneath it. Concentrate on it for a few periods of clarity. It may take a few minutes and you may be able to shed some tears. It is likely that you will experience moments of clarity where you clearly see the row in clarity. The eyes may feel slightly tight. The tears will occur as you try to accomplish this. If you are able to maintain that crystal clear image the greater improvement you'll see. This can be difficult to accomplish the first attempts, but as you work with it, the more easy it becomes and will enable you to view smaller and smaller texts throughout your improvements.

Myopia: Summary of how it can be reversed

Stop using all but lenses in all of your daily tasks. When possible, do not use these lenses when this level of correction is required.

If prolonged working in close proximity is needed then use reading glasses or plus lenses. Move to a sufficient distance so as to reduce the blurring of text.

Add bright light to your work and reading space since this can naturally enable your eyes to be more clear

Make sure you spend more time in well-lit outdoor spaces and constantly focus on objects in the distance.

Chapter 10: Good Habits For Vision

Similar to other lifestyle adjustments like dieting or exercising making good eye-healthy practices requires a slight change to your routine to allow for to achieve. Once you have learned the best way to overcome myopia it is important to ensure that your vision is sharp by staying away from behaviors that lead to poor vision initially.

Have a pair or glasses to read with at all times until you have clear vision

As long as your vision remains normal, it is best to stay away from work areas that are not protected by being protected by the "protection" of reading glasses. If you're seated near your desk or reading material, and the text is sharp and simple to read it is likely that you're not close enough. Make use of reading glasses.

While reading close-up ensure that the text is sufficient distance that it causes a slight blurring, whether using reading glasses or by shifting the text away from it enough to cause the characters appear slightly blurred. Make sure you have a pair glasses close by and wear them when you're looking at something that is closer to your blur.

If you're just starting to get your sights back, they could appear blurred that instead of putting on reading glasses, just take off your corrective lenses since this will cause enough blur. If you improve then you'll need to put on reading glasses or else it would be necessary to sit on a very far away from the material you work with.

If you're hoping to accelerate your progress You can put them on for the entire every day. This is a great method to get quick, visible outcomes.

Avoid using your existing corrective lenses

The restriction of the usage of your lens may not be the best choice dependent on work schedules or other obligations. But, it's one of the most effective strategies to regain your sight.

The use of prescription lenses only the point of necessity, and only for extremely short durations. The harm done to your vision was resulted from the excessive use of prescription lenses which were worn without a need.

Develop your eyes to view more clearly

It is essential to put in efforts to keep your eyes in top shape. What is the most common thing that occurs to those who suffer a fracture to their limb and have to put on a cast in order to allow the bone to recuperate? The body is unable to utilize these muscles on that area of their body. As it is, the muscles weaken or become much smaller and weaker due to the lack of exercise.

In the case of the eyes of yours, you have be able to utilize them in the way they were designed for originally. Eyes are designed to allow you to look up close, from and all distances between. The key is to make efforts to make use of your eyes to their fullest capacity. Even though we may have to stay in doors at all hours of the day doesn't mean that we can only utilize the eyes at close ranges. The eyes can be suffering from the symptoms of cabin fever when they're within the same space for many hours. Take a break from the home and take them out for a look around at distant objects. One of the easiest things to do is take a stroll. It's a great reason to get away from your daily routine.

Utilizing both the near and far sides of your vision will allow your eyes to experience a greater scope of focus. Utilizing corrective lenses over the years has led to the eyes to be able to concentrate only on distances that are close, and it is necessary to repair this harm.

Make sure to take frequent breaks during your near your work

Take frequent breaks. If you're working at your computer for the entire day be sure to stop each 20-30 minutes and take a look around at things like trees or birds far away. If you're in the middle of reading The same principle applies. Make sure to take frequent breaks. This can reduce eye strain as well as improve your eyes' ability to concentrate.

If possible you can take your book outdoors. Outside reading will ensure you've got sufficient lighting, provided that there's not a solar eclipse, or any other conditions that cause dark outdoor lighting.

Make sure you spend as much time outdoors as you can in light. Light-colored environments enable people to see easily and accelerate your improvement.

It is a good idea to take a look at objects in the distance and attempt to get them in focus.

If you're trying to train your eyes to concentrate, they are likely to change. They'll adjust to any situation you put them in. They have adapted to the use of prescription lenses, and they change size and shape. In trying to focus your attention on objects in the distance and making the eye see clearly, you're allowing your eye to change.

Chapter 11: Prevention

With the means to correct myopia, you're likely seeing some improvements. What can you do to make sure that you keep the progress you've already made and keep the condition from getting worse? How do you keep the improvements? After putting a considerable amount of energy and time making your health better You don't intend to regress. This chapter will focus on the steps you can take to keep the progress you've made is in the right direction: away from excessive diopter. We will look at ways we make sure that will be lasting. can last for the long haul.

1. Prevention

We learned from previous studies, there's an important correlation between the amount of the amount of time that is spent indoors reading and the incidence of myopia. There are a few strategies are available to help prevent myopia, specifically among children.

If you have to temporarily wear lenses that correct your vision, do not wear them in close proximity to your work.

If you're at this point it's possible that lenses for correcting your vision are about to sound awful. This is because they're. They should be accompanied by the warning labels to stop misuse.

Keep adhering to your good eye practices

If you've made substantial improvements, you'd like to revert back what you've made, don't you? That means adjusting your life style to make sure that you keep up with your vision health.

What other things can be done to keep myopia from becoming worse?

Naturally, we are spending some hours indoors. However, when you're reading, working on or browsing your smartphones, be sure you are in a well-lit surroundings.

Make sure your indoor area includes excellent lighting

Insufficient or poor lighting can make the task of seeing and to read. If you're in the dark studying or working, it is a good idea opening your blinds or curtains so that the maximum amount of sunlight be reflected. This is the most effective type of light that you can get. Alternately, you can use high-quality desk lamps that light your reading or working area. This can allow the reader to read at an extended distance than you had not the same brightness. It is possible to test this with a smartphone. The brightness can be turned completely down, and observe how far you are able to read with no text blurring. After that, you can turn the brightness all the way. Then, you will be able to read the text, but at a considerably greater distance.

Get outside and enjoy the sun

Like we said earlier the exposure to sun is useful in helping to prevent and reduce myopia. Be sure to get plenty of daily time. Develop a routine to get outside for walks at the most beautiful period of the day. appreciate the natural world. Consider pursuing the outdoors as a pastime that can encourage you to get out more frequently.

A lot of work in the near area without reading glasses can be dangerous and could make your eyes increasingly myopic.

Reduce this exercise as often as you can. If you are unable to do it, attempt to break frequently.

2. Maintenance

Reading glasses can help prevent any adverse effects from performing the work in a hurry and may assist in the process of an "tune-up".

If you are feeling like you're spending working in the office then you should be more attentive when using your reading glasses.

You can wear the glasses for several hours during all working day (not solely for close work). If you are wearing them for an extended period of time while you do any task that's not related to work, you will notice an increase in vision as you take them off. This might not be terribly obvious, but frequent use is a good "tune-up" to keep your eyes functioning properly.

If you choose to wear them throughout the day long, make sure you are cautious on the streets! The plus lens can alter your vision a bit, which means it is more susceptible to slip on the stairs such as.

Use a stronger plus lens. The majority of people don't have an adequate plus lens. They see slow improvement and may have difficulties in achieving clear vision.

Human body is amazing in its capacity to heal and adjust. The eyes are not any more or less resilient. If you are wearing +4 lenses initially, your eyes might struggle to read, making difficult for you to work normal. But, give it time and you'll be amazed by the effect can have on improving your vision in just 3-4 hours.

Adjust your lifestyle in order to stay clear of circumstances that can result in myopia

Maintaining your eyesight is about changing your life to the point where it is possible to stay away from actions that could create myopia.

Avoid dimly illuminated indoor areas.

Observe good eye habits

"Look 20 feet when you are outdoors

Do your practice with distant vision regularly, and look at objects on the edge of the horizon

What are you able to do in the winter months if you reside in an area that doesn't not see a lot of sunlight?

The seasons can have an effect the lives of those living closer to the equator, or in a place with a lot of sun-filled days have an advantage. What can you do during winter even if you're in an area that is dark?

If you reside in a place that is characterized by only a few hours of sunlight the best option is to improve the brightness of the indoor space.

Other obligations at work and personal can limit your time in a position to take a walk even during those brief hours of daylight when sunlight is plentiful lighting, and even bad weather can hinder you from taking a walk.

So, it's vital to have consistent light and brightness in the indoor space. It is possible to benefit from buying more powerful lamps or investigating other lighting options.

Make sure your eyes are tuned up

When you've made enough progress to see 20/20, yet you are finding that your eyesight may be weakening it is probably due to poor vision routines. It is possible that you have become accustomed in reading even though you're seeing clearly. It is natural to draw whatever you're doing or reading closer to the eye. It is natural to lean into and flex your neck. Be careful not to do that and make an effort to avoid this. The reading material should be moved further from you.

The most effective approach for now is to conduct an update on your vision. The solution is easy. Wear an extra lens that is strong for all day and continue with your everyday activities. Do your best to bring blurred objects to the center of your vision, and they'll gradually appear clear. Be very cautious moving around in particular going either up or down the steps.

The result should enhance your vision a little after a few hours. The more you use them, the quicker your eyesight will improve.

As with maintaining a automobile, changing oil as well as scheduling adjustments are essential to ensure the best performance. In winter, especially when the days are diminished and we are spending much of our time in a dim surroundings, and it's even crucial to ensure you follow good practices to prevent myopia from increasing.

If you're looking at your mobile for a long time each day at too short to a distance, you can reverse your course. These things happen within your reach therefore you don't require any visual corrections to do these things. If you believe that it's impossible, keep in mind that as time passes you'll be able that you can do it with the naked eye.

These aren't distant activities. Therefore, if we are unable to go out due to weather conditions or different reasons, we must keep an eye on our health. But, wearing lenses while working on computers as well as while using smartphones must have enough power to keep from the deterioration of your eyes.

It's not a good idea to wear reading glasses while you brush your teeth. But it could speed up your progress by using it more frequently.

If you are aware of the methods to stop the development of myopia, it is evident that the same techniques are applicable to prevent it. If I look back the first time I had glasses on I'd like to have learned about these strategies.

If your kids are about to enter classes and schools It is the ideal time to recommend adopting healthy eye-sight habits in order to prevent myopia from the beginning.

In the event that nearer the time there will be an obvious decline in vision, it could be corrected by beginning using reading glasses while using books. Regular usage of reading glasses can aid in preventing vision loss due to excessive work, which is often the prevalent in modern society.

Chapter 12: A The Nearsighted Crisis

The World Health Organization (WHO) classified the condition of nearsightedness, also known as myopia, as a worldwide problem. The organization predicted that in 2050, approximately five billion people which is about half the global populace, will be nearsighted. The number was forecast prior to the epidemic in 2020. Naturally, the magnitude and number of these numbers will be significantly higher because of the duration of the stay-at-home prescription.

Nearsighted people are unable to perceive clearly from a distance however, near vision remains clear based upon the level of nearsightedness. A condition that is nearsighted could lead to severe eye conditions including bleeding in the retina, retinal detachment excessive pressure in the eyes, macular degeneration cataracts, or even blindness. Everyday increasing numbers of young youngsters are being placed in closesighted (minus lenses) glasses, which can increase the severity of this condition more quickly than it has ever been. Children who are as young as five old are now wearing -1.00 nearsighted glasses, whereas just several years ago older children between the age 10 to 15 years old were wearing that type of prescription.

It is possible to ask why youngsters require nearsighted glasses in the first place or even why parents must be concerned. The reason lies in the notion that the more young the child diagnosed with the condition and the more quickly this problem gets worse. A lack of proper nutritional intake for proper eye development and continuous stress on the fragile eyes, improper using prescription eyeglasses as well as the inability to detect the indicators of a slowing eyesight loss are among the main reasons for the alarming rise in cases of myopia across the globe.

Actually they could have an eye prescription of -5.00 or even more. The vision can be compared to vision that is based on light, which means seeing the blurred light and dark images, with no help of any lenses that correct the vision. When faced with an disaster, such as the occurrence of earthquakes or fires the children don't have the functional vision needed to keep them out of harm if they should get their glasses damaged or lost. Along with causing a an everyday burden for these patients, this issue also causes a significant financial burden on the individual, state as well as the government level. Therefore, significant measures must be taken to stop closesighted prescriptions from becoming a problem. If your child is showing indications of diminished distance vision, the most effective treatments should be administered promptly to prevent the prescription for nearsightedness from escalating.

Parents are fully aware of the "bad habits" that their children exhibit that can cause poor eyesight. But, they'd be amazed at how fast and detrimental these routines result in. The children may be able to see 20/20 in the office of a doctor and after two months of summer, you could see 20/200. It's about -2.00!

Using Digital Devices Too Early and Too Soon

We should begin at the youngest age at which those infant eyes are "trained" to become nearsighted. We often see children as young as two years old or less - holding and focusing on their iPhone or iPad in the supermarket, restaurant or even in the doctor's waiting room. They are using electronic devices at a too young age and too fast! The eye structures of these children eyes and dedicated ones aren't equipped to handle the intense tension and strain caused by the brutal use of long-term close-viewing. Because of this in the same way that nature intended that it adapts itself to view clearer and better at close distances and will lose clear vision when in distance. When you look close for long periods of time, the quality of vision at distances decreases.

The initial sign is your child's eyes narrow while looking up at clearly visible distance images. Squinting can help in clearing the distance image for a brief period of duration. If this continuous tension on your eyes is not stopped, vision will get worse, and the prescription will grow. As prescriptions increase the risk of serious eye issues are likely to begin developing. One of the best ways to stop the use of digital devices with our kids is simple and straightforward to state, to not give them access to the device. Parents must be taught to avoid giving those electronic devices that require charging their children for use as "toys." One important note for parents to remember is to be sure to never "play" on their iPhones their own devices. Instead, they should return to basics with toys that do not cause eye damage, but also engage the brain. These include Puzzles Legos as well as sensory/tactile balls as well as bead mazes.

Not enough lighting Protecting against Myopia Development

One of the key elements that play an important influence on the growth of nearsighted/myopia is light. The majority of children are forced to sit on a computer or iPad for the majority during their working days. This is not only straining the eyes of children, but it doesn't allow the children with enough time during the daytime to get outdoors to exercise and enjoy lots of sunlight exposure. Many studies have proven that sunlight exposure from natural sources can play a vital role in slowing the growth of myopia.

An investigation conducted in Denmark revealed that sunlight plays a role as a key element in myopia, a condition that affects many people. Based on this study it is clear that due to the absence of sunlight during the winter months, children in school are prone to developing myopia rapidly. The incidence of myopia growing during summer is lower than during winter. The light wavelengths create the retinal dopamine reaction Dopamine is a neurotransmitter responsible for controlling the growth of the eyes. A person with a high nearsightedness has an eyeball that's elongated. The size of the eyeball will be larger when compared with those who are not nearsighted. So, a walk when there is natural light can "strengthen" the eyeball and help all children.

Improper Nutrition for Optimal Eye Development

Our society is the age of "microwave" society where everything must be completed quickly. Unfortunately, we have shifted away from the traditional way of life and our families seldom eat home-cooked meals or fresh picked from the farm and veggies. Spending the time with family to enjoy meal together is an uncommon moment. Fast-food or microwave cooking has drastically reduced our nourishment for the development of our children's eyes. Fast-food, the high consumption of sweets, microwaved and frozen foods are the children's regular meals. Thus, necessary steps must be taken in order to supply children with enough nutrition and nutrients they need for efficient and healthy eye function. The most nutritious foods include omegas, antioxidants as well as nuts and seeds.

Constant, Non-Stop Stresses on Delicate Eyes

If we were to do a weightlifting exercise over a long amount of time, without taking it go, what would be the result for the muscles? They'd begin to feel pain, and could even get into severe muscle spasms. As muscle spasms develop they cause the muscles to become stiff or stiff. The muscles would become stuck in the same position.

What happens if had to sit and read or make use of our eyes on computers, iPhone, or iPad for long periods of time without blinking or having a break? Our eyes' muscles could experience muscle spasms. Eyes become "stuck" in that one posture, which is the near-seeing one. Eyes don't show discomfort, however there could feel some discomfort. Eyes of children are strong. They aren't aware of the discomfort or pain; which is where the threat is. There's no signal for kids to quit looking at their eyes when they are in the distances they are too close to. So, a continuous stream of use on digital devices put continuous stress on our fragile eyes. Eyes adjust to close-up vision, and distance vision gets decreased. So, blinking and stopping frequently to look at a distance are essential in order to keep a balance between near and distance vision in order to maintain a the balance between the various distances.

Inappropriate Eye Devices That Worsen the Condition

The act of reading isn't natural. In nature, we're hunting. Our eyes were originally developed to hunt in search of food. After that, the written word was created. We believe today that learning and reading from books is the key to our survival which is why we're trying to accelerate the development of our kids as fast as we can. The toddlers learn the alphabet by using the iPad to learn the recognition of numbers and letters. It's unnatural for eyes to focus on close the distances they see for too far away. As soon as we think about, their vision for distance will becomes blurred. If your child starts to use nearsighted/minus-lenses eyeglasses, the prescription will start on a path of prescription increase year after year. It is therefore imperative not to let them follow the same way. Legos, building blocks Legos maze games, and building blocks are among the most enjoyable activities available in this age. When a child begins learning the alphabet, the best type of glasses include compensated lenses. They are an eyeglass with a lower plus that will help to relax the eye system, reducing tension when working with your eyes when you are at close distances. However, frequent breaks are required in order to stop muscle spasms occurring during close-range distances. This strategy can help ensure clear, 20/20 sight for the child.

Ignoring the Warning Signals of Oncoming Eye Deterioration

If you're reading this book with your hands, there is a chance you or someone else you know has nearsightedness. Many research studies has revealed that 80% to 90% of Asian descendents have nearsightedness. Asian adolescents are not the only ones affected However, the condition has begun to become more frequent among teens from all ethnicities and races. The likelihood of a child developing nearsightedness is very significant. So, parents have to keep an eye attentive to any signs of the condition. Computer use habits must be taken care of. Regular breaks should be planned within the home. Utilizing tips, tricks, and the methods described in this book will provide the best weapon to stopping myopia from developing and preventing.

Chapter 13: The Nearsighted Eye Doctor

My Perfect Vision

My birthplace was Saigon, Vietnam. My early years were straightforward. The school day was a regular routine at night, then we would play outside of the house, along with everyone else from the nearby neighborhood. Played until it became too dark for us to observe any thing. It was time to go to bed and the day would repeat itself exactly as it did over and over again. My daily routine was straightforward and relaxed and I was blessed with perfect vision.

After that, we quit Vietnam. My family moved to Germany. The climate was so cold, it was impossible to play outdoors. My free time was filled with a new love of reading. I was a constant reader and read through all my free time. I completed one book one after the next. I do not remember ever stopping reading. In my ignorance I had been "training" my eyes to develop myopia.

From 20/20 to 20/400

I was a total nerd reading every day for many years. I had no idea about the fact that my distance vision was not very good. It was my belief that everybody had this kind of vision. I did not even question my vision. When I was sixteen my family relocated to America. We had gorgeous conditions and could venture out to play in the sunshine. At this point, I had developed a unhealthy habit of being indoors constantly as well as, you guessed it studying. Also, it was at this point that I was able to pass the test for driving and also my vision exam. Why did I pass this test? It is likely that I have learned to squint and utilizing that technique to pass the vision test.

Aware of the Worsening of My Eye Condition

After passing my driving test, I took my buddies to the cinema. While driving to the theater, when I turned to the left, at an intersection I heard the sound of a crash. Then, I fell unconscious for about a minute. After waking up the next morning, my car was destroyed. It was gone! I realized my vision was weak enough that I could not even notice the approaching car when I turned to the left. Following the crash My dad drove me to see an eye specialist. The doctor said my vision was 20/400 with a the prescription being -3.00.

Finding the Solution & Implementing It for Success

Unfortunately, I believed that I'd always depend on glasses in order to be able to see clearly. When I graduated from the high school level, my father recommended that I be an eye physician to assist children learn to protect their vision so that they do not experience the same negative incident that I experienced. Even to this day I'm still awestruck by the impact the eye doctor can have for their patients' lives. We have a lot we can accomplish. It is possible to use our expertise and abilities to maintain the eyesight of people and ensure that they keep their eyes healthy for the rest of their lives. However, it is crucial that preventative treatment begin earlier for us to be able to defeat the scourge of myopia effectively.

I'm extremely blessed! I was able to attend an optometry program that is focused on two of the strongest methods for myopia control: orthokeratology and vision therapy. In the first few weeks of attending the school for graduate studies I was placed into therapy in order to discover techniques to preserve my vision. Additionally, I started Ortho-K therapy, which allows me to clearly see 20/20 while simultaneously learn efficient methods to stop my nearsightedness from growing.

Enjoying Continued Clear Eyesight

I was provided with two most potent tools I'm sure, which I use in my field and I have benefited immensely from these tools.

Vision therapy helped me learn the correct ways to utilize my eyes to have a comfortable and clear sight, and Ortho-K therapy helped me be able to see clearly in close distances and in the distance without having to wear lenses or glasses for daytime lenses. As time passed, these methods reduced my nearsightedness by -3.00 to -0.50! It's hard to believe but I am now able to enjoy the clarity of my near and distance sight, as I have done been for a long time, with no the necessity of using Ortho-K lenses. It is due to the techniques, tips and treatments which we'll discuss more in future chapters of this book.

"Dr. Vuong Would it be possible to offer her my eyes?"

When Karen was seated in the exam chair, I walked around to see her mother in the quiet room. I commanded her to sit in the chair on my left. I sat down and looked at Karen and requested that she look at some of the letters projected onto the wall. Karen was unable to read any of the letters. Therefore, I continued to increase the letters' size. In the end I showed her the largest letter in the chart: 20/400. She inquired "Are these letters? They don't have even see any letters. I can only see dark lines." She had her glasses on! After a few seconds, her mom was crying! After just a couple of minutes of crying and crying, she asked me an inquiry I thought I'd never have to. Karen's mom asked me "Dr. Vuong Is it possible to offer Karen my eyes?"

Karen's prescription has increased from the time she was four years old. My mom told me she was constantly using her iPad. As a ten year old she was -4.00. Following today's exam, we learned that Karen has a weight of -8.00. Mom was feeling so guilty she questioned me about it. I told her we'd take every step we can to ensure that her prescription is maintained and closely monitored her to ensure that it doesn't grow as fast than it did been in the past. It is a difficult task to put Karen onto Ortho-K lenses as -8.00 is too much of a prescription to ensure a good results in terms of vision. Naturally, the mom and daughter both were extremely emotional after they realized they did not intend to look after her.

After presenting them with all the advantages and disadvantages that Karen's Ortho-K program and they were pleased that I had the courage to commence Ortho-K treatment for Karen. Fast forward three years, Karen has been coming to us every month in order to receive training about the best practices and tips to maintain her eyesight. Her prescription has stabilized over the past 3 years. Their dedication and faith in us has resulted in this remarkable result. It wouldn't have been feasible if they didn't realize the risks of the condition of nearsightedness. They were aware of the dangers and took all the necessary steps in order to preserve and protect Karen's eyesight.

Chapter 14: The Essential Habits For Optimal Eye Health

The chapter will provide practical therapy techniques that are easy to incorporate into the daily life of your child. The discussion will focus on the definition of eye training. I will present a Near Far Hart Chart. It's among the most popular eye-training exercises, which is very effective at relaxing eyes all entire day. The course will offer tips on relaxation, breathing and visualisation in order to release the tension that children feel during the countless hours they study. Sitting in the correct position will be covered and the importance of regular breaks based on the 20/20/20 Rule. It is our primary rule of our office. I reiterate it to every patient at an Ortho-K health checkup. I am confident that all of them can easily repeat the phrase without doubt; they know it exactly what I say.

According to the American Optometric Association, up to 80 percent of pupils' education is via visual. In putting everything into view, as 80 percent of the information our youngsters have to be "uploading" into their brain comes through their eyes first which is a good reason to conclude that the vast majority of information is processed through the brain-eye route. So, having the fundamental skills for learning could help differentiate between a struggling child as well as academically proficient in the school years of critical importance.

Eye Training Therapy

A specialized area in our field that is specialized in providing efficient visual abilities for patients to develop or increase their basic visual abilities. It improves your visual comfort, ease and effectiveness, which is why it is known as vision therapy. It is comprised of regular in-office sessions and at-home therapy. In order to accomplish the goals of the book, which is to ensure that your child's eyes are at ease and to reduce the risk of them developing nearsightedness, I selected easy and easy eye-training techniques that can accomplish this goal. It is highly recommended that you use this technique every day for four hours - afternoon, morning, evening and prior to the bed. It is possible to do this simultaneously when you are eating breakfast and lunch or dinner as well as before you go to bed.

Near Far Hart Chart

The aim of this exercise is to enhance flexibility the distance and near by relaxing eyes muscles.

Print and attach your "Far Hart Chart" to the wall, the eye level, between six and eight feet from it (or set it in a position where is clear to you).

Print and grasp and hold the "Small Hart Chart" with your left hand. Utilize your left hand to put your right eye in the shade. Remember that this technique trains the both eyes at the same at the same time.

1. When your child is sitting or standing 6-8 feet away from the wall make them carry the "Near Hart Chart" in the palm of their hand, at an the level of their eyes, approximately forty centimeters off from his/her eyes.

2. The next step is to take a look at your child's "Near Hart Chart," and will read the alphabet from the left. The letter is "O." The letter O must be well-defined.

3. Have your child go through your child's "Far Hart Chart" and take a look at the"O" letter "O;" breathe in and out, and then relax while watching the letter "O" in the distance "O." Make it evident before returning to"the "Near Hart Chart."

4. Reread your "Near Hart Chart" and make your child take a look at the letter to right side of "O." This letter is "F," and the"F" is the letter "F" should be clear before turning their eyes towards"F. "F" at far.

5. Make the exact near-far eye movements as you read both the close and far word. Be sure to breathe deeply and let your mind relax.

6. Try to help your child keep a steady pace that reads one second for each alphabet.

7. When your child has completed the first letter across, continue the procedure for the left eye.

8. Ask your child to take the first line of a letters with the right eye.

9. After that, let your child go over the next letters with their left eye. Change back and forth between two eyes after each letter in the line Looking both ways.

10. The entire process should last around two to three minutes.

11. Do the exercise every day, 4 times per day to ease tension and strain over your child's eyes.

12. It is important that your child expands their peripheral (side) vision in order to be able to see further. As an example, when looking at the"O" letter "O," have your child take a deep breath and let it relax. they will realize that he or she can see additional letters on the right (or left) and the letters "F," "N," "P," "V," "D," "T," "E."

Breathing, Relaxing, Visualization

After examining patients with nearsightedness over the past twenty years, I observed that the vast majority have a similar trait. Nearsighted people tend to be extremely successful, and possessing the personality of a Type-A. This means that they are likely to experience constant stress. This could be because these are people who have high expectations for them or that their parents pressure them to do better from an early stage. Therefore, it is important to eliminate the pressure and anxiety which can be a key influence on myopia's development and progress.

When we get up in the morning, often unknowingly our bodies begin to tighten up. As a substitute, before we get up from bed or even before opening our eyes, keeping our eyes shut, make sure to take the deepest breath. Breathe all the air you can as feasible. While we inhale slowly then raise our eyes to look at the sky. Keep in mind that you do this when your eyes remain shut. There will be a feeling of height as if that you're being lifted into the air. In this instant, imagine that you are flying through gentle clouds. Feel just as light as the air. Feel present, and be aware of the oxygen that flows throughout your mind. Inhale slowly and drop your eyes from an upward angle to the lower position just like a balloon dislodged every ounce of air it could and let go of all worries. It is certain that you'll be having a fantastic day this morning. When you exhale, you can relax and then lay onto your couch and you'll feel the relief of relaxation and you will see a smile spread across the entire face. You are sure to be having a fantastic day today. Do this three times a day. This effective breathing technique, calming practice, and meditation practice will help set you or your child up to have a peaceful next day.

A proper sitting position guides the eyes to see clearly. Imagine that your body represents the top of the tower, and your eyes the light bulbs that illuminate the opening. If there were a lighthouse along the shore of the ocean the lights of our lighthouse would be bright, radiating outwards towards the ocean's open. What would happen if the lighthouse were situated on uneven ground? Aren't lights scattered out in all directions, without any focus or proper goal? So, in order to be able to study effortlessly you must be sitting in the correct position.

Here are a few suggestions for a proper sit position:

1. The the height of the desk for your child must allow the feet to be directly on the ground. If the desk is too tall then use a small stool to serve as you can use it as a footrest.

2. Check that your child can comfortably rest his or her elbows and both arms on the desk. Also, ensure the child is in a straight position, not being a slough.

3. Make use of a towel that has been rolled up or small pillows for support of the typical low back when you are on the computer or doing research.

4. The monitor on the computer should be between 18 and 24 inches from your child's face. Check whether the level of your child's eyes are around 15 degrees over the monitor of your computer. Your child is likely to be looking at the computer from a distance.

5. Practice the Sight-Saving 20/20/20 Rule.

One of the most simple rules to be aware of is 20/20/20. Intentionally observing this rule can help you maintain your 20/20 vision. Every twenty minutes you spend working on computers, studying a book or focusing your eyes on nearby tasks, focus your eyes for a period of twenty seconds, focusing your eyes from a 20 feet. Note 20/20/20 in the fridge or on mirrors in the bathroom or right in front of your computer. While we have frequent breaks at intervals of twenty minutes in a twenty-second period, watching the distance from twenty feet, it gives our eyes the flexibility to see both near and far. This can help in alleviating the daily strain that can be a burden on the muscles of the eyes.

Over the last twenty years I've kept reminding all my patients, nephews and nieces to follow this principle every each day. Everyone of our Ortho-K patients at my practice have the 20/20/20 rule at the heart. In every 20 minutes spent working in the vicinity (reading or using a computer, iPhone, iPad) you should take a break of twenty seconds with a focus on an area of about twenty feet. Patients should look towards the trees or cars speeding across the highway and breathe slowly in and out to ease tension. Patients practice this constantly for several years. Every year, when patients go for their annual complete eye exam the majority of them maintain their prescribed. The nearsighted prescription of their patients doesn't increase from year to year. I am pleased to say that a most of the patients maintain the excellent habits of study and work to adulthood, successfully stabilizing their vision and stopping myopia from growing. Don't be tempted to take the 20/20/20 lightly to save your eyesight from degrading!

Chapter 15: The Critical Eye Companions

What do you think you would take in case you had in a battle? What weapon, or protection gear should you ensure that you carried at all times? If you were wearing the right safety from a bulletproof vest body armor, could it be the difference between life and death? What would you do when I said that any protective eye equipment that your kids use for learning, reading or even computer usage could mean an impact on healthy or eye problems? This is an important fact to keep in mind and follow through in making sure your kids use them regularly. Make sure your kids carry the protective equipment with them throughout the day like they're the best of friends and partners. These are compensation glasses. What is the best way to Blue Light Blocker Lenses be used in conjunction with the compensatory eyeglasses in order to enhance the comfort of your eyes while studying working on a computers? How do we integrate all of these with the powerful companions with UV protection and lens that are impact-resistant to ensure kids' eyes are secure throughout the day? We'll discuss this detail in this section.

What are the best ways to ensure that Compensation Lenses help protect you from nearsightedness?

Between the ages of 2 to 3 years young children already use their eyes without control and in a hazy environment for hours at a period of. Naturally, we don't recommend that children utilize all electronic devices until they are have reached a certain age; usually when they reach the age of 9 or 10. We do understand that kids need to learn the alphabet. Instead of exposing them to the risk of poor eyesight, why not teach them the importance of glasses that protect against superheroes and dangers around the workplace (computer iphone, iPad,)? Set a standard that your child wear these Sight-

Protective eyewear whenever they work with any electronic device. This is your first line of protection against strain on the eyes.

From the age of three old, bring your child to the eye doctor who will recommend relaxing or compensation eyeglasses to your kid. Relaxing or compensation lenses are prescription lenses that have a low price. They're also referred to as readers. The lenses that are low could vary from +0.50 up to +1.50 or more, based the needs of the patient. The eye doctor in your area will be the most knowledgeable person to assist you in the best prescription for your child based on the examination of eyes. Then, ensure that your child undergoes their vision exam at least every six months and not annually. The short time frame can to guide you in understanding the condition of your child's eyes and make sure you address any problems necessary early rather than rushing into "repairing" it when it is too late and the prescription is excessive. I've witnessed that parents stare at me like they were stunned, after having realized that their children couldn't even read the large letters "E" of 20/400 size. Many mothers even broke down crying! Set out to watch out for any indication of poor or weak eyesight.

What are the advantages of using Blue Light Blocker Lenses?

The digital devices, fluorescent light as well as TVs emit blue-violet lights (within the 415--455 nm wavelength). The term is usually used to describe blue light. Blue light may create oxidative stress on the retina, which is the tissue layers that line the rear part of our eyes. The use of a computer screen for prolonged period of time could cause headaches dry, red, eyes or tired eyes, stiff necks. These symptoms are referred to as digital or computer-related eye strain, or Computer Vision Syndrome (CVS). Blue light can impact the quality of sleep a person gets. A prolonged exposure to high-energy blue light may impact the health of the retina and macula, causing them to get older prematurely. The flickering light can also contribute to a poor sleep pattern among the majority of teenagers.

One way to combat this is to use blue-light blocking lenses or blue-screens that also provide anti-glare shields. Limiting exposure to blue light could boost or sustain a normal evening melatonin levels. Better quality sleep may be obtained. People who wear blue light blocking glasses have reported less eyestrain, and less headache.

If you combine low prescriptions with blue-light anti-glare lens Computer vision disorder (or digital strain) can be greatly reduced. This will increase your levels of comfort while using your computer. A key point to computer users is to work on their computer for more than an hour prior to bedtime, as the use of computers can disrupt the quality of our sleep patterns.

(rapid eye movements) sleep. The REM stage is that occurs during the deepest phase of our sleep which allows us to get the best rest during our sleep. Utilizing electronic gadgets for a long time, and at night, they can affect the sleeping pattern. The ability to work and study could be harmed.

Powerful Combination for All Waking Hours

From the time my children were three years old I began to guide them down the path of protecting their eyes to protect them for the rest of their lives. One of the most effective options you can offer your child wear throughout the day is progressive lenses. What exactly are progressive lenses? It is possible to think that these lenses are only for mature individuals, and they are. The lenses were designed for those who require clear distance and near vision. Distance and intermediate (computer) and close glasses prescriptions are integrated to form one. As you gaze or feel the lens's surface it is difficult to see any distinction between the various prescriptions that have been merged into. Another kind of lens that is suitable designed for adults are bifocal lens. They come with a top part to allow for distance and a bottom part for near-prescription They do feature distinct lines through the lens.

We'll look into the reason at the reasons why progressive lenses are efficient in protecting your children from the development of nearsightedness. I began putting my children's wearing these lenses as early as the age of 3 because that was when at which they began to master the alphabet. If we offer children Bifocals they could be irritated by the line that appears that is in front of them and will be reluctant to wear these lenses. On the other hand, I provided my children lenses that were progressive with no prescription for the top of the lenses as well as a prescription for a low plus at the lens' bottom. I explained to them that these lenses are like a eye protectors, as they guard them against negative things that could happen. Additionally, the lenses have blue-light blocking as well as a low prescription, and an anti-reflective coatings to block the glare that enters the eyes of patients. The lenses are constructed of polycarbonate lenses which are impact resistant. When something lands in the eyes of the wearer, these lenses will act as shields that are shatterproof. The lenses also have UV protection. They also were changed into sunglasses as my kids played outdoors. These powerful lenses have helped to protect my kids' eyes and those of my patients from any unwelcome increase in prescription and shielded them from dangerous UV radiation, as well as hazardous objects aimed at the eyes.

Only 3-5 Families Accomplish This

My private practice was established at the age of my children, which was very young.

At the age of three and a half, I gave the progressive lenses with anti-reflective coating, low plus in transition, blue light blocking lenses. Also, they learned in this early age to utilize the 20/20/20 rule in conjunction with the various vision treatments that are described in the book. Presently they are both at college as well as in high school. After having closely followed their prescriptions and thoroughly, I am delighted to see that one of them is prescribed -0.50 and the other is able to see perfectly.

If I ever see parents bring their three year old baby to the clinic, I would tell them the story of my kids. I explained to them the way I managed to do it, and how it is working to stop the nearsighted lens from growing and maintaining perfect eyesight for my kids. I informed them that right now is the perfect time to start keep their eyesight in good condition since they aren't on to develop nearsightedness. I provided them with all the tricks, tips and exercises for the eyes. I also informed my students that despite the fact that I've been practicing for more than 20 years, and instructed thousands of parents on the best ways to ensure perfect vision especially for infants Only 3-5 families have been able to complete the task.

What can I do to be sure? We provide free vision screenings. Following our eye exam and screening, we arrange for all our younger patients with 20/20 vision for a visit to our eye clinic at the end of three months, six months nine months, as well as one year. It might be a shock to you. In the 3rd month The majority of patients showed signs of progressing towards -0.50 nearsightedness. After six months, they're around -1.00 and from there. The rate of progression towards nearsightedness increased afterward in an uncontrolled way. Perfect, natural eyesight wasn't possible anymore. The observation may be unusual of different optometric methods. My practice is near the middle of the highly Vietnamese and Chinese population.

What is the chance of this happening even after spending more than 30 minutes reviewing the entire details? The same thing happened after I had warned the children that, after every year of practicing I have only seen 3 families who return with 20/20 vision. Most of them are slowly seeing their prescriptions creeping up over time and is increasing each year. This is why research has shown that over 90% of Asian youngsters are nearsighted. I've seen this phenomenon for a long time. There are a myriad of reasons that contribute to the rise of nearsighted prescriptions for Asian youngsters. While I am adamant about that this is a good practice the parents usually believed that their children had good eyesight for granted. They believed that electronic devices could be dangerous in this short time. When these children become nearsighted the progression will be rapid in the absence of drastic measures implemented. The majority of parents believe that the most appropriate option in this case is to introduce them to an Sight-Saving Therapy of Ortho-K. We'll be discussing the highly efficient treatment in the following chapters.

Chapter 16: Work With You're Vision Therapy Coach Along With You

What would be wonderful to have your child's or her own personal vision therapy coach on hand throughout the day? I see the abilities and the information I share into my students to be an integral component of a fantastic education which your kids can carry everywhere they take them. It is my belief that children to be able to complete specific tasks, they must be enjoyable and engaging. Engaging children in the decision-making process of the instruments we employ gives them a confidence and conviction of taking care of their eyes. Engaging them in choice making process regarding what's best for their eyes is crucial.

The most important thing is to teach children about the advantages of having eye health. Explain that it is important to keep the eyes "fit" by taking good treatment of them everyday. Have your kids ask "What kind of sports would you choose to play if you had great eyesight?" It is also possible to tell them, "You can enjoy the fireworks on Fourth of July or New Year's Eve with healthy and clear vision." In this chapter, you'll discover how to keep your child's Vision Coach accompany you at all times once they've mastered the techniques of uteri-zing the standard analog clock as well as the rule of 20/20/20. In addition, we'll teach them to use the Palming as well as Acupressure Points to ease the tension of everyday life and encourage healthy eyes.

The Clock Can Reverse Nearsighted Condition

Many homes were equipped with wall clocks. Today, we mostly make use of our phones to keep track of the time. There are however many advantages to keeping a wall clock within your the home. In addition to allowing clocks to beautify your house to look stylish and classy, but they also aid in the health of your child's eyes. This eye exercise helps relax and boosts blood flow to the eyes muscles. The clock should be approximately twelve inches wide that is hung up on a wall that is about ten feet or a place where your child is able to be able to see the numbers as they gaze upwards during the time of homework. The clock you need is an analog clock with the hour, second and minute hands. the clocks.

Applying the 20/20/20 rule encourage your child to gaze upwards at the clock following each ten or twenty minute period of work. Slowly change the focus between twelve o'clock and one at a time, then two, after which three o'clock. Continue to move clockwise each hour, until the child returns to 12 clock. Encourage your child to take a breath and calm down before moving your eyes gently between twelve o'clock and 11 o'clock, then 10 o'clock. Do this clockwise every hour, until they return to 12 clock. This will take less than 30 minutes.

In doing this, the exercise achieves two key aspects. The circular movement of eyes relieves tension, improves flexibility and the circulation of blood to the eyes. If you do not own the luxury of a wall clock and you are looking for a new one, it is enjoyable to look with your kids for one. Let them choose the style and color that they'd like to glance at throughout the day as they work at their laptop or doing their homework. The design will stand out in the room, and they will feel happy that they chose the color for their personal eye training to protect themselves from the growing problem of myopia (nearsighted).

Palming and Acupressure Points Can Release Eye Tension

It's a great idea to have kids and parents engage in all of the Acupressure and palming exercises in a group. Before we begin working with the acupressure points in the eyes, it is necessary begin the first process of palming. Palming is a straightforward efficient, easy, and convenient method to keep a clear sight. You can do it anyplace and takes just about 2 or 3 minutes. Relax your neck and shoulders the palms of your hands for approximately 20 seconds or until hot. Put your palms on your eyes. Let the warmth of your palms relax your eyes and muscles surrounding your eyes. Take a deep breath and exhale slowly, allowing yourself to enjoy the moment. While closed in your eyes, envision yourself standing on top of the mountain, with fresh air refreshing, slightly cool and rejuvenating.

Acupressure

Eye muscles feel excessive tension this can result in an insufficient flow of blood to that region. Acupressure is a great treatment that helps ease the strain in these regions in which blood flow may be obstructed or stopped.

Based on the wisdom of the ancient Chinese medical theories, there are invisible energy lines which flow throughout our bodies. These lines are known as meridians, also known as Qi/Chi. Acupressure massage can be a beneficial method that relieves tiredness with the intention of removing blockages, which can create chronic pain as well as other health concerns. The application of gentle pressure to the meridians by using thumbs, fingers or even palms. Massage of these points on the local area may relieve pain and discomfort. A healthy balance is maintained by the body's lymphatic system and the circulatory system aid your body's immune system to be able to self-heal its own self.

My nearsighted patients have headaches post their school days. There are many possible factors that cause headaches. It is my preference for patients to see their physician at home to rule out any other possible factors. Most of the time, patients suffer from an increase in nearsightedness over time. Alongside various treatment strategies I typically suggest acupressure to the eyes.

I selected three easy and simple acupressure methods to use up to 4 daily. The exercise should take less than 2 minutes.

Around the Eyes

Imagine that your child has to participate in a game. The animal they depict is an animal called a raccoon. In the presence of the raccoon's eyes your head, and using your pointing fingers Move those fingers in the eyes closed in the same way you would draw a circle of black or the letter "O" around them. Then, slowly move the fingers using a slight force on the eyes, and then cover your eyebrows as well as the lower lids in the circle. Once you're finished If you placed black ink on your fingers, you'd be able to see a large black circle that circles your eyes. It's like the eyes of a raccoon. Your fingers should be moved around your eyes 3 times in clockwise direction and 3 times clockwise. This could help using coconut oil or massage oil to your fingertips. Make sure you breathe in a slow, steady way while relaxing your shoulders and neck muscles to improve your vision. It will ease the eye muscles and increase the flow of blood oxygen and, consequently reduce tension in the eye muscles. It is an easy and effective way of preventing the build-up in "bad blood" and muscle spasms, which could lead to eye problems.

Between the Eye; The Invisible Third Eye

Check your eyebrows. There's space between the eyebrows. Make use of either or both of your index fingers and gently press the middle between your eyebrows. This is right above your bridge of your nose. Close your eyes and the area you want to massage, also known as"the "third eye", for around two to three minutes with a short circular movement. Massage oil is a good choice and be sure to breathe slowly and inhale. Relax your shoulder and neck muscles. By massaging these muscles, you can reduce redness, fatigue, and eye strain.

Along the Side of the Nose Bridge

Many people blow their noses and then place a napkin in front of their nose and using both their fingers pointed towards the nasal sides. When they have blown their noses, they wash their nostrils making use of both pointer fingers while squeezing their nostrils, and then pushing the napkin down.

Then, keeping that movement in your mind, apply both index fingers to place one index finger on the other nostril's side. In lieu of blowing out your nose out, gradually and slowly massage two sides of your nose bridge at the same time. With a circular motion use your fingers to move across the sides of your bridge towards your forehead. The relaxing massage should last between two and three minutes. Do this at least three times per each day, in between studies. It helps alleviate sinus headaches and nasal congestion.